OPTIMUM
NUTRITION
BEFORE, DURING AND AFTER
PREGNANCY

About the Authors

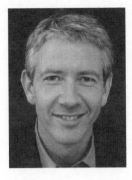

Patrick Holford is a leading light in new approaches to health and nutrition. He began his academic career in the field of psychology. While completing his bachelor degree in Experimental Psychology at the University of York, he researched the role of nutrition in mental health and illness, and later tested the effects of improved nutrition on children's IQ – an experiment that was the subject of a *Horizon* documentary in 1987. He became a student of twice Nobel prize winner Dr Linus Pauling, who believed that the future of medicine was 'optimum nutrition'.

In 1984, with the support of Dr Pauling, Patrick Holford founded the Institute for Optimum Nutrition (ION). A charitable and independent educational trust for furthering education and research in nutrition, ION is now one of the most respected training colleges for clinical nutritionists. At ION he pioneered many radical ideas in nutrition, from the importance of antioxidants to the dangers of HRT.

He has written over twenty popular books, now translated into seventeen languages. The first, *The Optimum Nutrition Bible*, has sold over a million copies worldwide. Backed by more than twenty-five years of research and clinical experience, Patrick Holford is convinced that good health starts in the womb and even before conception.

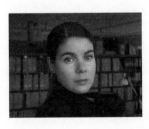

Susannah Lawson, DipION, is a health journalist and practising nutritional therapist. She trained at the Institute for Optimum Nutrition and also with the pre-conception care charity Foresight, for whom she is one of their accredited practitioners, helping couples overcome fertility problems naturally. She combines writing and research in the field of nutrition with seeing clients at her busy practice in Hampshire.

patrick HOLFORD
& Susannah Lawson

OPTIMUM NUTRITION
BEFORE, DURING AND AFTER
PREGNANCY

THE DEFINITIVE GUIDE TO A HEALTHY PREGNANCY

piatkus

PIATKUS

First published in Great Britain in 2004 by Piatkus Books
Reprinted 2004, 2005 (twice), 2006 (twice), 2007 (three times)
This edition published 2009 (twice), 2011, 2013, 2014

A CIP catalogue record for this book
is available from the British Library.

ISBN 978-0-7499-2469-0

Typeset in Berkeley by Phoenix Photosetting, Chatham, Kent
Printed and bound in Great Britain by CPI Group (UK) Ltd, Croydon, CR0 4YY

Papers used by Piatkus are from well-managed forests
and other responsible sources.

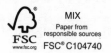

MIX
Paper from
responsible sources
FSC® C104740

Piatkus
An imprint of
Little, Brown Book Group
100 Victoria Embankment
London EC4Y 0DY

An Hachette UK Company
www.hachette.co.uk

www.piatkus.co.uk

Contents

Acknowledgements

The first version of this book was co-written in 1987 by Patrick's first wife and mother of his children, Liz Lorente, during pregnancy. Patrick and Liz learned a lot raising two healthy kids and working with many mothers-to-be. We are immensely grateful to her for her role in this pioneering work. Since then there have been many breakthroughs in our understanding of the essential role of nutrition during pregnancy, and we are indebted to the many pioneers whose research we have called on for this version. Among these are Professor David Barker, Professor Derek Bryce-Smith, Arthur and Margaret Wynn and Professor Michael Crawford. We are especially indebted to Belinda Barnes, the founder of Foresight, for her inspiration and tremendous dedication; to Fiona McDonald Joyce for her help with recipes and food ideas; to all the couples and mothers we advised and quizzed on real life as a parent; and, finally, thanks to our partners Gaby and Matthew for putting up so patiently with our long hours of writing.

Patrick Holford and *Susannah Lawson*

Guide to Abbreviations and Measures

Most vitamins are measured in milligrams or micrograms. Vitamins A, D and E are also measured in International Units (IUs), a measurement designed to standardise the various forms of these vitamins, which have different potencies.

1 gram (g) = 1,000 milligrams (mg) = 1,000,000 micrograms (mcg)
1mcg of retinol (1mcg RE) = 3.3 IUs of vitamin A
1mcg RE of betacarotene = 6mcg of betacarotene
100IUs of vitamin D = 2.5mcg
100IUs of vitamin E = 67mg

In each part of the book, you'll find numbered references. These refer to research papers listed in the References section on page 241, and are there for readers who want to study this subject in depth.

Introduction

❧

HAVING A BABY is the most incredible thing you can do. But creating a beautiful baby that will grow up healthy, happy and bright is down to more than luck or good genes. What you do before, during and after pregnancy (and especially what you eat) has the most profound effect. That's why we'd like you to know what you need to do to give your child the best possible start in life.

Your diet and nutrient intake can maximise your fertility (and the same applies for your partner), helping you to conceive when you want to, even if you're a first-time mother in your late thirties or early forties. You can also follow some simple steps to clean up your body – giving yourself a pre-pregnancy 'MOT' – to make sure you create the optimum environment for your baby to develop, as well as boosting your own health and wellbeing.

Once you're pregnant, we show you how to keep healthy and energised, and avoid many of the common problems such as anaemia, morning sickness and stretch marks. We'll also help you make sure your baby's getting all they need to develop perfectly, and tell you about supplements that can boost their IQ in the womb, plus reduce their chances of inheriting allergies or conditions such as eczema or asthma. Along the way, you'll learn about optimum nutrition and how to apply it practically to your life – not just while you're pregnant, but for the future too.

Why is all this so key? Because the vast majority of pregnancy problems are the direct result of sub-optimum nutrition. And although many people believe they eat a 'well-balanced diet', more than twenty years of clinical experience has shown us this is not the case. Birth defects, for example, are increasing, with one in sixteen babies now affected. One in four pregnancies end in miscarriage and 7 per cent of babies are born with a low birth-weight, which increases their risk of ill-health and disease in later life. The good news is now we know why, thanks to the pioneering research of people such as Professor David Baker from the Medical Research Council Epidemiology Unit at Southampton University, Professor Michael Crawford from the Institute of Brain Chemistry and Human Nutrition in London, and Derek Bryce-Smith, Emeritus Professor of Chemistry at the University of Reading, to name but a few. And we'd like you to know so you have the best chances of a healthy pregnancy and a super-healthy baby as a result.

As making a healthy baby doesn't stop after the birth, we show you how to continue optimally nourishing your child through breast feeding, weaning and up to the age of five. We also offer help and advice for tackling common problems during this first stage of life – from nappy rash to broken nights, fussy eaters to frequent infections, plus how to best approach the emotive area of vaccinations. Throughout, we include lots of recipes and ideas for healthy, delicious food to whet your appetite and inspire you in the kitchen. You'll see for yourself that the optimum nutrition approach not only makes scientific sense, it tastes good too!

We hope you enjoy the journey and wish you a healthy pregnancy and a happy baby to show for it.

Patrick Holford and *Susannah Lawson*

PART ONE

∽

YOUR PRE-PREGNANCY MOT

'I want to be a great mother. Where do I start?'

Ideally, before you get pregnant. Although pregnancy is a natural event and can frequently come as a surprise, if you're still in the planning stages, making sure you – and your partner – are in the best possible condition will greatly increase your chances of having a healthy, happy and problem-free pregnancy with a healthy baby at the end of it.

In this section, you will learn about preparing your body for pregnancy, including:

- How to maximise your (and your partner's) fertility.
- Making your womb a 'pollution-free' zone.
- The truth about drinking, smoking and passive smoking.
- How to virtually eradicate the risk of birth defects.
- Why a low 'homocysteine' level is your best guarantee of health.
- How to banish allergies and boost your and your future baby's immunity.
- Why increasing your essential fat intake now can give you a super-brainy baby later.

CHAPTER ONE

∾

Maximising Your Fertility

WHEN WE SPEND so much of our lives trying to avoid getting pregnant, it's natural to assume that conceiving is a piece of cake. Often it is. But sometimes it isn't, as the many couples we've seen in our clinics needing help demonstrate. However, we know that if you get yourself ready by following the basic steps we outline here, you'll dramatically increase your chances of getting pregnant when you want to, and will end up with a healthy baby. For a woman, what you do in the month leading up to conception, when you are maturing that auspicious egg, is the most critical. For the man, it takes up to four months to make new sperm from scratch, so they have to be good for a little longer! (More on that in the next chapter.)

Fertility and the speed of conception depend on many factors – some psychological, some physical, some nutritional and some environmental. For example, conceptions are very high during holidays since stress has a major impact on fertility. Knowing how to time sex to coincide with ovulation (where the female egg is released to be fertilised by the sperm) also greatly increases your chance of conceiving. But most of all, your nutrition, especially your vitamin and mineral status, plays a crucial role.

It has been estimated that only one in twenty people in Britain genuinely receives adequate amounts of all vitamins and minerals to meet the European 'recommended daily allowance' (RDA). However we personally don't even consider these 'RDA' levels to be optimum. Practically everyone we see in our clinics display signs of deficiency in at least some if not many of the key nutrients. But while a diet lacking in all you need may not actually make you infertile, it could make you 'sub-fertile' and reduce your chances of getting pregnant. A marginally fertile woman trying to have a baby with a man with a low sperm count, for example, may not be able to conceive.

So anything that can be done on either side to improve fertility increases your chances of getting pregnant when you want to and also increases your chances of having a super healthy baby. You don't just need to be fertile. You need maximum fertility.

Hatching healthy eggs

Unlike men – who produce a regular supply of fresh sperm after puberty – women are born with all their eggs (or ova) in place. Your ovaries contain about two million eggs at birth, but, as you age, they gradually disintegrate. By puberty, there's about 750,000 left, and by age forty-five, only 10,000 can be left. Your fertility is dependent on the health of these eggs and your reproductive organs, plus your body's ability to produce the right balance of hormones to 'mature' your eggs ready for ovulation with each monthly cycle. Getting the right mix of supporting nutrients is key to this.

In this section, we identify specific vitamins, minerals and fats that can make you more fertile. However, no nutrient works in isolation. Eating a well-balanced diet enhanced with supplements that boost levels of all essential nutrients is the best route to achieving good health and maximising your fertility. This is more specifically outlined in the Better Pregnancy Diet and Supplement Plan in Part Two, as this is the programme we've found works best not only during pregnancy but also before.

Tune up your sex hormones

The mineral zinc is absolutely vital for reproductive health. Infertility, low sex drive and period problems have all been linked to inadequate levels. Together with vitamin B6, zinc affects every part of the female sexual cycle. Working in partnership, these two nutrients ensure that adequate levels of sex hormones are produced. For example, one hormone called LHRH (luteinising hormone releasing hormone) causes your pituitary gland to stimulate the development of an egg (or ovum) that causes ovulation. A deficiency in either zinc or B6 causes a deficiency in LHRH, so your fertility decreases.

Adequate levels of zinc and B6 also increase your desire for sex (which is why zinc-rich oysters are called an aphrodisiac) and alleviate pre-menstrual problems – women who suffer from premenstrual syndrome (PMS) are often zinc deficient.[1] After conception, zinc and B6 ease pregnancy sickness and post-natal depression, as well as increasing the chances of having a healthy baby.

Oysters, lamb, nuts, egg yolks, rye and oats are all rich in zinc, while B6 is found in cauliflower, watercress, bananas and broccoli. The optimum intake is 20mg of zinc and 60mg of B6, which you can achieve with a diet that includes these foods (see page 110 for more sources), plus a good multivitamin and mineral supplement (more on this in chapter 12).

Why the right fats are essential

Fat is an important part of our diet. But while the wrong kinds of saturated fats – found in processed foods, meat and dairy products – are rich in most people's diets, the right kinds of fats are normally lacking. Oily fish such as mackerel, herring, sardines and salmon are rich sources of one kind of essential fat called Omega 3. Nuts and seeds are rich in the other kind – Omega 6 (see 'The fats of life', page 76, for more on these). Like zinc and B6, Omega 3 and 6 fats are needed for healthy hormone functioning, so a deficiency is likely to affect your menstrual cycle and therefore your fertility.

To make sure you get enough essential fats, aim to have a portion of oily fish two to three times a week and eat a handful of fresh, unsalted seeds every day. Seeds are also rich sources of minerals (including zinc) and protein, so they make a perfect snack. But because of their fat content, they are prone to damage when they come into contact with oxygen (a process called oxidation – see below). For best results, follow our magic formula: keep a mixture (50 per cent flax and 50 per cent pumpkin, sunflower and sesame) in a screw-top jar in the fridge, then grind a heaped tablespoon in a coffee or food grinder each day to sprinkle on cereals, yoghurt or soups. Grinding releases their oils and makes it easier for your body to absorb the nutrients.

Limit the impact of ageing

Although oxygen is essential to life, it also causes damage – and reproductive organs are particularly sensitive. When oxygen is broken down in our bodies, highly reactive molecules called free radicals are formed, and these harm, or oxidise, other molecules, which can start a chain reaction of damage. For example, when an apple is cut and comes into contact with oxygen in the air, it gradually turns brown on the outside and begins to rot. The same would happen inside our bodies were it not for a complex repair system that minimises damage. However, this system is dependent on a good source of 'antioxidant' nutrients from our diet. If these are lacking, then we age faster, are more prone to developing disease and can become less fertile.

So, to keep your body young, you need a good intake of antioxidants. The main antioxidant nutrients are vitamins A (both the animal form retinol and the plant form betacarotene), C and E, plus the minerals zinc and selenium. Phytonutrients are a recently discovered class of antioxidants – bioflavonoids and lycopene are two you may have heard of. These enhance our absorption and utilisation of other antioxidant nutrients as well as having protective qualities themselves, and are often responsible for giving a plant its colour, which is why eating a 'rainbow' selection of fruit and vegetables ensures you get a good variety of phytonutrients. Essentially, they all work together to protect your body and especially your reproductive organs. Studies have shown that both vitamin C and vitamin E boost fertility in women and men,[2] while vitamin A is needed for your ova to grow and develop before ovulation. However, a word of caution. While the betacarotene version of vitamin A is perfectly safe, too much of the animal form, retinol (found in fish and animal liver), can cause problems (see page 120 for more on this), so get the lion's share of your intake from vegetable sources.

The best sources of antioxidants

What to include in your diet to slow down ageing and protect your reproductive organs.

Vitamin A (betacarotene) – Carrots, sweet potatoes, dried apricots, squash and watercress.

Vitamin C – Green vegetables, peppers, kiwi fruit, tomatoes, citrus fruits and berries

Vitamin E – Nuts, seeds, oily fish, avocados, beans and sweet potatoes

Selenium – Brazil nuts, sesame seeds, tuna, cabbage and whole grains

Zinc – Meat, fish, oysters, seeds, nuts, eggs and green leafy vegetables

Phytonutrients – Fruits and vegetables of all colours – red beetroot, blueberries, orange apricots, yellow peppers, pink grapefruit and green leafy vegetables

The Better Pregnancy Diet and Supplement Plan in Part Two outline exactly how to incorporate the right balance of antioxidant nutrients (see chapters 9, 10, 11 and 12). This programme will not only help to ensure a healthy pregnancy, but will also enhance your fertility and aid conception.

Protect yourself from 'anti' nutrients

Anti-nutrients are substances that deplete your body of vital resources while contributing nothing nutritionally themselves. Refined sugar can be classed as such because it contains no nutrients of its own yet uses up stores of vitamins and minerals as your body processes (or metabolises) it. But anti-nutrients that have a greater impact on your fertility are those that actually damage your body – alcohol, cigarettes, drugs and environmental toxins.

- Alcohol: When you are preparing to conceive, drinking any alcohol at all can reduce your fertility by half – and the more you drink, the less likely you are to conceive.[3] One study showed that women who drank fewer than five units of alcohol (i.e. fewer than five glasses of wine or two-and-a-half pints of beer) a week were twice as likely to conceive within six months compared with those who drank more.[4]

- Tobacco: Unsurprisingly, smoking hampers fertility too. In a recent study at the Institute for Reproductive Medicine in Germany, researchers have found that smoking damages the quality of eggs in ovaries, reducing the number capable of producing a baby.

- Coffee: Sadly, you can't even seek solace in a cup of coffee. Research has shown that caffeine – also found in tea, chocolate and cola drinks – decreases fertility. Just one cup of coffee a day can halve your chances of conceiving.[5]

The increased number of chemicals and pollutants in the environment is also a factor (see 'The great British sperm disaster' in chapter 2). And toxic metals such as lead and mercury can play havoc with your fertility as well as damaging a developing baby – these are outlined in more detail in chapter 3.

Weight matters – fertility decreases in both obese and skinny women

Infertility rates go up in times of food shortage – because without sufficient nutrients, a woman's menstrual cycle will stop. But in our resource-rich Western world, thankfully this doesn't happen – unless the food shortage is self-imposed.

Slimmers and underweight women run the risk of becoming infertile if they don't eat enough to maintain a regular menstrual cycle. Swedish research has revealed that the 'average' woman (i.e. 5ft 4in/1.60m of medium build) will stop having periods at 8st 3lb (52kg).[6] But even if you are underweight and still have periods, your diet can affect your fertility.

We've seen women who've become infertile as the result of combining a low-fat diet with constant exercise – even though they are having regular periods and 'appear' perfectly healthy. As a result of extensive research, fertility expert and Harvard professor Rose Frisch maintains that only 10 per cent of women are fertile with a body mass index of 18 (see box, page 10). She says: 'Many women who maintain body shape made popular on the catwalks throughout the world are completely infertile.' This is because your body needs a sufficient intake of fat (albeit the right kind) to produce the hormones required for ovulation.

Likewise, if you are overweight, your fertility can be reduced. Even moderate obesity – classified as a body mass index of 25–30 – reduces your chances of conception and increases the risk of miscarriage.[7]

So, for maximum fertility, you need to eat enough of the right kind of fats and be neither under nor overweight. As each of us has an individual bone structure and body shape, there is no definitive answer to what your normal weight should be, but the body mass index is a useful guide.

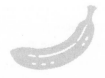

The body mass index

The body mass index (BMI) is a popular method of measuring weight in relation to height. You can determine yours by following this formula:

Divide your weight in kilograms by the square of your height in meters.

For example, if you weigh 62kg (9st 7lb) and are 1.70m (5ft 7in) tall, your BMI is

$62 \div (1.70 \times 1.70) = 21.5$.

Below 20 is considered underweight, 20–25 normal and 25–30 overweight.

Heal hormonal imbalances

A common factor in women who are overweight is a hormone imbalance. As well as sex hormones, our body produces hormones that control the way we metabolise and utilise food. You will probably have heard of the hormone insulin – this escorts glucose, the breakdown product of carbohydrate, out of our blood (after it's been absorbed from our digestive tract) and into our cells, where it's used to make energy. Insulin therefore regulates blood glucose. But many people have difficulty balancing their blood glucose – sometimes they produce too much insulin and their blood glucose level drops, causing fatigue, irritability and stimulant cravings (i.e. for sugary foods, chocolate, coffee or cigarettes). Others have cells that become 'deaf' to the message insulin's giving them, so the glucose stays circulating in the blood and then gets repackaged by the liver and stored as fat. These people therefore put on weight easily.

Poor blood glucose control is also a factor in polycystic ovary syndrome (PCOS), which is a common cause of infertility thought to affect one in ten women. As the name suggests, this condition causes multiple (poly) cysts to form on the ovaries where eggs mature but don't actually 'hatch'. This means there's no egg released for fertilisation.

As well as a tendency to being overweight and having problems controlling blood glucose (i.e. energy levels), other symptoms of PCOS include excess body hair, acne, mood swings and having erratic or few periods. The conventional treatment is to prescribe a type of contraceptive pill that reduces excess testosterone (another contributory factor) and regulates periods. However, if you are trying to get pregnant, being on the Pill is not an option. The nutritional approach is to help correct underlying imbalances, reverse the symptoms and restore fertility with a programme that, among other things, swaps refined carbohydrates and sugar for wholegrains, and more fruit and vegetables, and reduces intake of saturated fats from meat and dairy foods while increasing essential fats from oily fish, flaxseed and nuts – basically, the programme outlined in the Better Pregnancy Diet and Supplement Plan in Part Two. Also see the section on homocysteine, page 12. And for more on how to address more complex cases of PCOS, read Dr Adam Carey and Collette Harris's excellent book, *PCOS: A Women's Guide to Dealing with Polycystic Ovary Syndrome*.

Another common symptom of hormonal imbalance that affects fertility is endometriosis. Usually caused by producing too much oestrogen, this can also be helped by nutritional therapy. Dian Shepperson Mills, who trained with Patrick at the Institute for Optimum Nutrition, is an expert in this field and has written, with Mike Vernon, *Endometriosis, a Key to Healing Through Nutrition*.

Is too much stress reducing your fertility?

Stress is an everyday fact of life in the twenty-first century. But when you're trying to conceive, too much can reduce your fertility and play havoc with your health. Our reaction to stressful situations is the same today as it was in early stages of our evolution, when we had to be primed to 'fight or flight' to ensure survival. If we came face to face with a fierce predator, all our energies would be diverted into running away or protecting ourselves rather than producing reproductive hormones or digesting the food in our gut. Although we are unlikely to face such dangers today, we still respond in the same way when we have a pressing work deadline, get stuck in traffic or have to juggle too many responsibilities. And as these sorts of events occur daily, some-times hourly, bodily systems like reproduction and digestion can become neglected. Stress also uses up stores of nutrients – especially B vitamins – which are crucial for a multitude of functions, including fertility.

We know that being relaxed boosts fertility because holidays are a common time to conceive. But for most of us, taking time off is lim-ited to a few times a year. The rest of the time, if you find it hard to relax, get irritable, are unable to 'shut off' from the events of the day or have trouble sleeping, stress is having a negative effect on your health – and this could reduce your fertility.

Shakespeare had a point when he wrote: 'There is nothing good or bad but thinking makes it so' (*Hamlet*, Act 2, Scene 2). Unless your house burns down or someone dies, most stresses are not disasters. Thinking they are, however, can easily overwhelm you. So if you feel you need help to address the way you react to stress, there are many options open to you. Learn to meditate, take up t'ai chi or yoga, create some 'me time', have a regular massage, learn positive thinking – whatever will help you to relax and get on top of stress. See the Resources section in the back of the book for useful contacts. The Bet-ter Pregnancy Diet and Supplement Plan will also provide all the nutri-ents you need to help your body cope better with stress.

Maximise your fertility by lowering your homocysteine

Homocysteine is a protein-like substance naturally found in our blood. However, a diet lacking in sufficient nutrients or a genetic impairment can mean that levels of homocysteine are higher than they should be, and this can contribute to all sorts of health problems, including infertility.

So significant is homocysteine in pregnancy that we've included a whole chapter on it (chapter 6). But if you're still in the planning stages, we believe it's vital to get your level tested now and, if necessary, reduce it with the right supplements and dietary measures before you conceive (full details in chapter 6). Not only can it boost your fertility, it will also help you avoid many of the problems that can occur during pregnancy.

Reducing your homocysteine may also benefit other disorders that can reduce fertility. For example, researchers from Italy have found that women suffering with PCOS are much more likely to have high homocysteine levels.[8] So as well as following a dietary programme to address the causes of PCOS, having your homocysteine tested and treating this accordingly may reduce the symptoms and therefore enhance fertility (again, see chapter 6). Once your homocysteine, or 'H score', is below 6 you are in the best possible condition to conceive.

Getting your partner tested may also increase his fertility. In men, high homocysteine is strongly associated with low sperm motility. Motility is the 'swimming power' of sperm, which determines whether they can make it to the egg and penetrate it, or run out of puff. In one study, high homocysteine was associated with 57 per cent less motility![9] This may be because the chemical process our bodies use to convert homocysteine to beneficial substances – a process called 'methylation' – is absolutely vital for healthy sperm production.

The silent sexual disease epidemic

Sexually transmitted infections and bacterial infections can greatly reduce fertility, or increase the risk of miscarriage and damage to your baby once you've conceived. Yet many would-be parents don't even know they are at risk. This is because some diseases, such as chlamydia, produce few easily detectable symptoms. As a result, doctors estimate that one in ten women under the age of twenty-five is infected with chlamydia and these women are unlikely to find out they have it until they investigate why they are having problems conceiving (chlamydia is now being cited as one of the most common causes of infertility). If you do manage to conceive while infected, it can lead to an ectopic pregnancy, miscarriage or premature birth. It can also infect your baby during birth, leading to conditions such as conjunctivitis, gastroenteritis, unspecified viral disease and failure to thrive.

Other asymptomatic bacterial infections classed as 'Group-B streptococci (GBS) and mycoplasmas' can also damage fertility as well as causing problems during pregnancy and harm to your baby. For example, GBS is the leading cause of meningitis and infection in newborn babies in the UK, yet the mother may not even realise she is infected.

Gonorrhoea also causes infertility and the number of cases diagnosed at genitourinary medicine clinics has risen every year since 1997. According to UK National Statistics, between 1998 and 2007 the number of cases in the UK rose by 42 per cent.

Urinary tract infections (UTIs) are also common, affecting 5–7 per cent of women during pregnancy. If left untreated, they can also cause mental retardation in babies.[10]

So, even if you think you're in the clear, it's wise to get yourself and your partner checked out before you try to conceive. One British doctor conducting a preconceptual screening for couples following the Foresight preconceptual programme found that 69 per cent of his patients had one or more bacterial or sexually transmitted infection.[11]

Wannabe parents over thirty

More women are choosing to delay pregnancy than ever before – the percentage giving birth age 30 and over in the UK increased from 30 per cent in 1986 to 46 per cent in 2006.[12] Men, too, are leaving parenthood until later. The average age of first-time fathers has increased to 32, and around one in ten babies is born to a father aged 40 and over.[13] And while there are many psychological advantages to being an older parent, physically it can be much more demanding.

To begin with, getting pregnant is more difficult – after the age of thirty, the viability of your eggs starts to decline and you are likely to have fewer cycles in which you ovulate. A thirty-five-year-old woman takes, on average, twice as long to conceive as a twenty-five year old.

Male fertility – previously thought to be unaffected by age – also starts to reduce after the age of twenty-four. Researchers at the University Division of Obstetrics and Gynaecology at St Michael's Hospital in Bristol studied 8,500 couples and found that the older a man is, the longer it is likely to take his partner to conceive, irrespective of her age. The odds of conceiving within six months of trying decrease by 2 per cent for every year that the man is over the age of 24. 'It tells us that to some degree men as well as women have a biological clock that starts ticking as they get into their thirties,' says Dr Chris Ford, who led the study.

Older parents also have a greater risk of conceiving a baby with genetic abnormalities such as Down's syndrome. For example, the risk of a chromosomal abnormality in a woman aged twenty years is 1/500, increasing to 1/20 by age forty-five. But this is partly because your body has had more exposure to an unhealthy lifestyle (nutrient-deficient diet, smoking, drinking etc.), stress and pollutants. So taking care preconceptually and throughout your pregnancy can greatly increase your chances of having a healthy baby.

In fact, research has shown that under ideal conditions – if you are in good health with perfect nutrition, good antioxidant protection and limited exposure to pollutants (i.e. the programme outlined in this book) – the effect of age on the chance of achieving a successful pregnancy may be less than previous studies show.[14] Certainly, we are finding many older couples have healthy babies after adopting the optimum nutrition approach we prescribe.

Leave eighteen months between pregnancies

If you already have one or more children and are planning to have another, the length of time you leave between each pregnancy can have an effect on both your future health and that of your baby. Studies sponsored by the World Health Organisation show that having babies too quickly in succession slows down the rate at which your baby develops in the womb and that, after birth, this can lead to smaller stature and poor performance at school.[15] Other research claims that 13 per cent of low birth-weight babies and deaths before or just after birth are as a result of birth spacing that is too close.[16] And we've found in clinical practice that women who aren't optimally nourished before or during pregnancy have a far greater propensity to develop health problems, and these can impact on the health of their next child if they don't take time to restore nutrient stores before conceiving again. Growing a baby and giving birth is hugely physically demanding and you should give your body at least eighteen months to two years to recuperate before repeating the experience.

Choose the right method of contraception

As you prepare your body for pregnancy, it's wise to eliminate as many possible 'pollutants' as possible. The Pill can be classified as such because it depletes your body of essential nutrients, particularly B vitamins – of which the vitally important folic acid is one – and vitamin C. The Pill also increases copper levels in your body and high levels of copper have been associated with infertility and birth defects. What's more, too much copper can lower your zinc levels (because these two nutrients are antagonists of each other) and zinc is particularly key during pregnancy for the growth of your baby.

Stopping the Pill at least three months before you plan to conceive will help your body return to its natural menstrual cycle – so you become fertile again – and will give you time to redress any nutritional imbalances. While you are doing this, use barrier methods of contraception (i.e. condoms or a diaphragm). There are also natural family planning methods where you learn to identify when you ovulate, so can abstain from sex or use barrier methods on your 'fertile' days – usually for five days before ovulating and for two days after. Unlike the calendar-counting rhythm method, natural family planning uses a more scientific approach, which makes it much more reliable (see 'Knowing when to try', opposite). It's also useful to become aware of your fertile days so that when you're ready to conceive, you'll know the best time to try. See the Resources section at the back of the book for contacts that can teach you natural family planning.

Know when to try

Unlike the Pill or coil, natural methods of birth control do not interfere with the cycle of ovulation and menstruation. During your cycle – which can vary from twenty-three to thirty-five days – there is only one day in which an egg is available for fertilisation. However, sperm usually live for three days and under excellent conditions can survive for five. Therefore, if you know when you ovulate, having frequent sex in this five-day window dramatically increases your chances of conception. So, how do you find out when ovulation occurs?

The discovery that a different type of mucus is produced just before ovulation led to the development of the simplest and safest method of birth control. Unlike normal vaginal mucus, fertile mucus is sticky and thread-like – a bit like egg white. It's designed to nourish and protect the sperm, providing it with channels to move along, thereby greatly increasing its chances of reaching the egg.

In a World Health Organisation study, 90 per cent of women could identify their fertile mucus within the first month of learning what to look for. Another way to tell is by monitoring your resting temperature (i.e. as you wake up in the morning) – this will drop, then rise very slightly as you ovulate. There are also ovulation predicator kits that you can buy without prescription from chemists and large supermarkets. For more details, read *A Manual of Natural Family Planning* by A. M. Flynn and A. Brooks.

Once you're ready to get pregnant, being in good health at the expected time and shortly after conception is especially important. Catching the flu or a virus in the early stages of pregnancy can harm your baby and increase your risk of miscarriage, so if you become unwell while trying to conceive, abstain from sex until you have fully recovered. You can reduce the risk of getting ill in the first place by boosting your immune system. For more on this, read chapter 7.

Still having problems conceiving?

If, after following this advice, you still have problems conceiving, we recommend you see a nutritional therapist specialising in fertility (see Resources section), or contact Foresight, the preconceptual care charity, for a referral to one of their practitioners. These specialists can work with you and your partner to identify and try to correct any underlying problems such as polycystic ovarian syndrome (PCOS), hormonal insufficiency, parasite or bacterial infections, heavy metal toxicity and food allergies. And if you're planning to try conventional fertility treatment such as IVF (in vitro fertisation), they can also help you maximise the chances of it working successfully. However, Foresight's own research shows that a more holistic treatment gets the best results. While just 23.4 per cent of IVF treatments result in a birth,[17] Foresight achieves more than 78 per cent. In a Foresight preconception survey (1995–7), 1,076 couples (1,061 of whom had previous fertility or miscarriage problems) gave birth to 779 babies, and a further 67 couples were pregnant when the survey ended. Most of those who did not get pregnant did not complete the preconception treatment programme.

In summary, if you want to boost your fertility, start to adopt the following measures three months before you want to conceive:

- **Follow** the Better Pregnancy Diet and Supplement Plan outlined in Part Two (specifically chapters 9, 10, 11 and 12).

- **Eat** regular sources of the key fertility nutrients – in particular zinc (oysters, lamb, nuts, egg yolks, rye and oats), B6 (cauliflower, watercress, bananas and broccoli) and essential fats (oily fish and fresh, unsalted seeds).

- **Also** boost antioxidant nutrients – aim to eat at least five portions of different coloured fruits and vegetables a day, plus a handful of fresh nuts and seeds.

- **Supplement** a good diet with a daily multivitamin and mineral formula (see chapter 12 for more on this).

- **Reduce** sources of 'anti-nutrients', such as refined foods (anything made with white flour or sugar), alcohol, tobacco and caffeine, and limit exposure to or use of industrial chemicals and pharmaceutical drugs.

- **Learn** relaxation techniques if you're frequently feeling stressed.

- **Test** your homocysteine and if levels are high, aim to reduce them before conceiving.

- **Have** a sexual health check to screen for possible infections (many of which are asymptomatic).

- **Come** off the Pill at least three months before planning to conceive and learn natural family planning techniques that will then later help you know when you're at your most fertile.

CHAPTER TWO

A Man's Guide to Making Super Sperm

I N CASE YOU didn't know, it takes two to make a baby and it isn't quite as easy as just having sex. When you do it, how you do it, what you ate the week before and what you drank that night all have a direct effect on your sperm hitting the target.

In the past it has been wrongly assumed that the woman is responsible in the majority of infertile couples – yet up to 60 per cent of infertility is actually down to the man.[18] Men also play a large part in causing birth defects – defective sperm may account for as much as 80 per cent of genetic abnormalities. But this isn't new information. In the US, a survey of medical literature in the 1960s by Friends of the Earth found similar statistics and reported that: 'American men presently cause the vast majority of birth defects'. Given that one in every sixteen babies has some level of defect, and one in six couples fails to conceive at all, it is not only advisable, but essential for you to take some simple steps to make sure you have super-healthy sperm able to deliver the goods on time.

As sperm takes about four months to develop, preparing in advance for conception is just as key in men as it is in women.

The great British sperm disaster

The quality of sperm has dramatically decreased over the past 50 years or so – a review of 61 research papers published between 1938 and 1991 and looking at nearly 15,000 men found that overall sperm quality and density has dropped by 50 per cent.[19] In another study of British men born between 1951 and 1975, the concentration of sperm and total sperm number per ejaculate has progressively fallen by 2.1 per cent a year.[20] Today, in 90 per cent of male infertility cases, low sperm count is responsible.[21]

Diminished sperm count is a serious matter. Many animals produce up to 1,400 times as much sperm as is needed for fertility. In contrast, the average human male produces only two to four times more.[22] So what is going on?

The decline in semen quality has been attributed to environmental rather than genetic factors – that's an increase in pollution, unhealthy lifestyles, stress and poor nutrition. For example, smoking reduces sperm concentration by about 24 per cent[23] while alcohol is toxic to the male reproductive tract and can cause significant deterioration in sperm quality – in heavy drinkers it can result in complete infertility.[24] Heavy and sustained smoking and drinking also depletes the body of key nutrients, especially B vitamins that are vital to reproductive health.[25] And coffee is bad news for men wanting to conceive. Studies have shown the higher the coffee consumption, the lower the sperm quality.

Increased sex is also part of the problem – abstinence greatly increases sperm concentration, yet today's man has more sex than his counterpart fifty years ago. But the most serious factor appears to be exposure to environmental chemicals that have 'oestrogenic' effects – that is they mimic the female hormone oestrogen. Not only are these associated with declining sperm counts, but also testicular cancer. And while most men don't believe they're in any danger, we encounter these chemicals every day – they are found in paint, plastics, food packaging, pesticides and cosmetics. So doing the decorating, eating food or drink that's been wrapped in plastic packaging, even using male grooming products, can impact on your sperm count.

Is your job making you infertile?

If you or your partner are exposed to chemicals in the workplace, this can have an even greater detrimental effect on fertility. A report by the Association of Scientific, Technical and Managerial Staffs funded by the Equal Opportunities Commission called *Reproductive Hazards at Work* identified those most at risk. These included workers in the textile industry, nurses handling some anti-cancer drugs and anyone exposed to certain dyes, solvents and weedkillers. For example, regular exposure to lead or mercury by metal industry and hospital workers or organic solvents handled by those working in laboratories, laundries, the textile and petrolchemical industries can cause reduced fertility and an increase in miscarriage, stillbirth and birth defects. Other studies have reported greater numbers of birth defects, including spina bifida and facial clefts, in babies born to fathers whose job involves exposure to agricultural chemicals, when compared to other occupations.[26]

Some prescribed drugs also have an adverse effect on sperm quality. For example, the drug susphasalazine, used in the treatment of bowel conditions such as ulcerative colitis, is known to reduce sperm count.[27]

Boosting male fertility

In practical terms, the first place for you to start is by avoiding coffee, alcohol, cigarettes and exposure to any suspect drugs or industrial chemicals for at least four months before you want to conceive. However, total avoidance of environmental chemicals is never possible, so improved nutrition provides an extra degree of protection.

Vitamin C, for example, has been shown to safeguard sperm from damage.[28] The importance of vitamin C for increasing fertility has been reported in a study in the *Journal of American Medical Association*, which showed that giving extra vitamin C increased sperm count as well as motility (this is the sperm's ability to 'swim' – which needs to be Olympian to have any chance of surviving the twenty-four-hour race up the Fallopian tube and arrive with enough gusto to penetrate the female ova). A group of thirty-five infertile men were given 500mg of vitamin C twice a day and their sperm tested. The results revealed 'continuous increases in percentage of normal sperm, sperm viability and sperm motility'. The most significant change that occurred to the sperm was a decrease in agglutination (the name given to the clumping together of sperm), which is associated with impaired fertility.[29]

Getting an adequate intake of essential fats is also important for male fertility. Essential fats are used by the body to make localised hormone-like substances called prostaglandins. Research has shown that men with poor sperm quality, abnormal sperm, poor motility or low count have inadequate amounts of prostaglandins.[30] The dietary recommendations are the same as those outlined for women (explained in more detail in chapter 11). But seeds are especially good as they are not only a good source of Omega 6 essential fats, but also high in vitamin E (particularly sunflower seeds). Vitamin E has been shown to increase fertility when given to both men and women.[31]

The mineral chromium is also an important nutrient, as a deficiency not only reduces our ability to make energy from the food we eat, but can also hinder the body's ability to make new cells, including sperm. Studies show that rodents fed on diets low in chromium have a significantly lower sperm count and decreased fertility compared to chromium-supplemented controls.[32] This mineral is frequently lacking in our diets due to the trend for eating refined grains and sugary foods that contain less chromium, while at the same time increasing our need for it. So swapping these foods for wholegrains and eating chromium-rich foods such as wholemeal or rye bread, potatoes, green peppers, eggs and chicken will help to boost levels, as will taking a daily supplement (again, this is outlined in more detail in the Better Pregnancy Diet and Supplement Plan in Part Two – you can follow the same programme as your partner).

The high rate of infertility in diabetics may provide us with another clue to the role nutrition plays in fertility. Diabetics are frequently low in vitamin A, which is essential for making the male sex hormones. Vitamin A can be found in both animal (e.g. liver, cod liver oil) and vegetable (carrots, sweet potatoes, apricots) foods. But it is also dependent on zinc to be properly utilised by our bodies.

Zinc for virility

Of all the nutrients known to affect male fertility, zinc is perhaps the best researched. Signs of zinc deficiency include late sexual maturation, small sex organs and infertility. A lack of zinc can also damage the testes.

In view of the fact that the average dietary intake of zinc is substantially lower than the recommended daily allowance (RDA), the effects of zinc on fertility may be quite substantial. A survey by the UK Ministry of Agriculture Fisheries and Food revealed that the typical daily diet provides only about 9.7mg compared to the RDA of 15mg.

Zinc is found in high concentrations in the sex glands of the male and also in the sperm itself. There it is needed to make the outer layer and tail and is therefore essential for healthy sperm. On a zinc-deficient diet, the zinc concentration in the testes falls to one-third the normal level.[33] As much as 1.4mg of zinc is lost with each ejaculation, so a prolific sex life and an inadequate diet would put a man at risk. In fact, in the nineteenth century many patients were diagnosed as having 'masturbation insanity' – perhaps the earliest suggestion of a link between zinc, sex and mental illness. (There may be more than an element of truth to the old saying that masturbation makes you blind and stunts your growth!)

As with women, zinc works with B6. Boosting levels of both these nutrients can increase male fertility.

In summary, if you want to boost your fertility, start to adopt the following measures at least four months before conception:

- **Follow** the nutrient-rich, wholefood diet outlined in chapters 9, 10 and 11 (i.e. the Better Pregnancy Diet).

- **Eat** regular sources of the key fertility nutrients – in particular zinc (oysters, lamb, nuts, egg yolks, rye and oats), chromium (wholemeal or rye bread, potatoes, green peppers, eggs and chicken), B6 (cauliflower, watercress, bananas and broccoli) and essential fats (oily fish and fresh, unsalted seeds).

- **Also** boost antioxidant nutrients – aim to eat at least five portions of different coloured fruits and vegetables a day, plus a handful of fresh nuts and seeds.

- **Supplement** a good diet with a daily multivitamin and mineral formula (see chapter 12 for more on this – you can take a similar supplement to your partner).

- **Reduce** sources of 'anti-nutrients' such as refined foods (anything made with white flour or sugar), alcohol, tobacco and caffeine and limit exposure to or use of industrial chemicals and pharmaceutical drugs.

- **Test** your homocysteine and reduce high levels before conception (see chapter 1 for more on this).

- **Have** a sexual health check to screen for possible infections, many of which are asymptomatic (again, see chapter 1).

CHAPTER THREE

~

Turning Your Womb into a Greenhouse

M AKING HEALTHY BABIES is like gardening. The best you can do is get the soil healthy, plant the seed, then feed and water it regularly. As you prepare to conceive, creating that perfect, nourishment-rich and pollution-free womb is the best birthday present you could ever give your baby to be. The research is clear. A mother's nutritional status at the time of conception, and in first few weeks that follow, is the single most important determinant of a baby's growth in those critical early stages.[34] So, more than at any other time in your life, your nutrition needs to be not just adequate, but optimum, if you want a truly healthy baby.

In the first two chapters, we focused on boosting your and your partner's fertility. In doing so, you're improving your health and therefore improving your chances of having a healthy baby. While we touched on reducing your exposure to harmful substances such as alcohol and tobacco in chapters 1 and 2, now we're going to look at potential pollutants in more detail and explain how you can prepare the optimum internal environment for your baby to develop in. You see, after nine months in your womb, your baby will be born largely complete, with all the heart, muscle and kidney cells he or she will ever have (as they grow, these cells can only be enlarged). And although the brain, nervous and immune systems will continue to develop, the infrastructure is already established prior to birth. That's why reducing your exposure to harmful substances, chemicals and pollution – and detoxifying what's already accumulated before you get pregnant – is important. Doing this will not only benefit the health of your unborn child greatly, it will also improve your own health, appearance and energy levels too.

Even among those clients we see who feel perfectly fit and well, we've found many are still deficient in key nutrients or harbouring toxins – and these can harm a developing baby. Unlike a fully grown adult, an unborn child is highly sensitive to the slightest changes in the supply of nutrients or indeed poisons. We know that while a woman may show no apparent sign of folic acid deficiency herself, such a deficiency can cause spina bifida in her unborn baby. Likewise, a woman with a high level of mercury or lead accumulated in her body tissues may appear reasonably healthy, but her baby could be born with physical or mental malformations. At no time is your child more sensitive and vulnerable than during their nine months stay in your womb.

Anti-nutrients in pregnancy

Good nutrition isn't just about what you eat; it's also about what you don't eat, drink or breathe. Many of the substances considered to be bad for us, such as alcohol, pollutants and cigarettes, cause their damage by interfering with essential nutrients. For instance, lead is a powerful antagonist to zinc and calcium, both crucial for mental and physical development. These anti-nutrients, perhaps not noticeable in tiny quantities in adults, can be dangerous to your baby.

However, it can be hard to distinguish between what is normal mental and physical development in a baby and what should be normal when we live in a world where the average person eats 14lb (about 6kg) of preservatives and additives, breathes 1g of heavy metals and has 1 gallon (about 4.5 litres) of pesticides and herbicides sprayed on their 'healthy' fruit and vegetables every year. Only when the effects of anti-nutrients such as lead pollution from petrol and chemical fumes or drugs such as thalidomide become truly dire do we do anything about it.

What is normal?

After discovering that high lead and cadmium levels and low zinc were associated with stillbirths, difficult pregnancies and deformed babies, Professor Bryce-Smith of the University of Reading began a comprehensive study to determine just how important these minerals are. He tested no less than thirty-six different minerals in a dozen different ways from a hundred mother and baby pairs. He measured hair levels, blood levels, amniotic fluid, placental levels, pubic hair, cord blood ... you name it, he tested it. Although his sample group all experienced 'normal' births (i.e. no complications or malformations), much to his surprise, their mineral levels were far from normal. He found that the lower the zinc levels in the placenta, the smaller the baby. Also, the higher the lead and cadmium levels, the smaller the baby. So clear were the results that Bryce-Smith can predict both birth-weight and head circumference just from analysing these minerals in the placenta. He also found a tendency for high aluminium levels in those who had premature placenta membrane rupture. Bryce-Smith's initial pioneering study was carried out in 1980 and the amazing results have led to many further studies, from which we can understand the dangers of anti-nutrients and the detrimental effect they have on pregnancy today. Let's take a look at what they are and then examine how you can find out if you're affected, and what you can do to protect yourself and your unborn baby.

Lead: reducing size and IQ

Birth-weight is a key indicator of health in later life. Research by Professor David Barker at the Medical Research Council Epidemiology Unit at Southampton University has found that the smaller the baby, the greater the risk of premature death from stroke and heart disease, for example. Bryce-Smith had already established from his work in the 1980s that the higher the lead, the lower the birth-weight. But a later study, conducted with Dr Neil Ward of the University of Surrey, found elevated levels of lead in the placentae of stillborn babies and those born with spina bifida or brain damage (hydrocephalus).[35] An American study also found higher levels of lead in babies who died of cot death.[36] Perhaps more interesting is the fact that this correlation exists even in mothers whose lead levels would be considered 'normal'. Like many environmental poisons, there appears to be no threshold at which lead can categorically be called safe.

Further evidence for the dangers of low-concentration lead has also been reported by child psychiatrist Professor Herbert Needleman. He found that lead levels recorded at birth correlate with intellectual development at age three.[37] At any age, lead is a powerful neurotoxin, but babies and children are particularly vulnerable as their brains and nervous systems are still developing.

Thanks to Bryce-Smith's pioneering work and his tireless campaigning, lead has been taken out of petrol. But although our exposure today may be lower than previous decades, lead pollution is still present in the atmosphere (it's even been found in the polar ice caps) and also comes from water contaminated by lead piping and from flaking paint and paint dust, pesticides, cosmetics and industrial exposure. When intakes of the essential minerals calcium, zinc or iron are low, lead becomes that much more toxic. Given that many pregnant women are deficient in all three, it's important to redress the balance through diet and supplements before you conceive.

Copper: why too much is bad news

Copper is both an essential element and a toxic one. Due to the widespread use of copper in water pipes, plus exposure from jewellery, kitchen utensils and even swimming pool anti-fungal agents, we are today more at risk from toxicity than deficiency. Of the 2mg we need each day, that amount is supplied simply from drinking water that has passed through copper pipes, irrespective of any copper that is absorbed from our food. What's more, long-term use of the contra-ceptive Pill, IUDs (intra-uterine devices) and fertility hormones such as Clomid further increase copper levels in the body. Yet high levels of copper depress zinc, which is vital not only during pregnancy (see page 110), but also for fertility (see chapter 1).

Once a woman is pregnant, the copper levels in her blood tend to rise dramatically and remain elevated for around a month after birth. The reason is believed to be because copper acts as a stimulus for the uterus. But if there's already a high level to start with, the additional accumulation can cause copper toxicity and this is far more common during pregnancy than at other times. In fact, too much too soon may be a factor in inducing premature babies or miscarriages.

High levels of copper may also be a factor in post-natal depression or mental illness. Copper depresses histamine levels in the body and since histamine is an important nerve transmitter this in turn affects the brain.

Mercury: a fishy poison

The saying 'mad as a hatter' originated because hatters used to polish top hats with mercury. And mercury, like lead, is extremely toxic. In elevated amounts it is highly teratogenic (literally meaning, 'monster-producing'). In the Minimata Bay disaster in Japan (1953–60) 111 people died and many more children were born with deformities after their parents ate fish contaminated with mercury leaked from a local plastics factory.

It's now known that mercury can easily pass from mother to baby via the placenta and a baby's blood can often contain up to 20 per cent greater the levels of the mother's, with four times as much concentrat-ing in the brain tissue.[38] As well as birth deformities, mercury can cause mental disorders, disturbed sight and hearing, digestive, kidney and heart disorders, immune dysfunction and hormone imbalances.

Sadly, due to widespread pollution, fish are one of our biggest sources of mercury. The larger and fattier, the greater the accumulation – up to nine million times the amount found in the water[39] – with tuna fish probably being the most contaminated. One in twelve American women of childbearing age has potentially hazardous levels of mercury in her blood as a result of consuming fish, according to government scientists.[40] As a result, the US Food and Drug Administration recommends pregnant women don't eat tuna, shark, swordfish or mackerel. And in the UK, the Food Standards Agency advises women who intend to become pregnant, or who are pregnant or breast feeding, to limit their consumption of tuna to no more than four medium-size cans or two fresh tuna steaks per week. It also advises avoiding shark, swordfish and marlin altogether.

Mercury is also found in water contaminated by industrial processes and in pesticides, but besides fish, our other most common source of this toxic metal is dental fillings. The mercury in teeth is not totally immobile and it's possible to detect traces of mercury in the breath of people with mercury fillings. After fillings have been fitted or removed, urinary mercury may also show a slight increase. Sweden has now banned mercury fillings for pregnant women, and although there is no such ban yet in the UK, it would be wise to have any dental work done a few months before you conceive or after you've finished breast feeding. And, even then, ask your dentist to use alternative materials to fill your teeth.

Cadmium: passive smokers beware

Like lead, cadmium can accumulate where zinc is low, and builds up in the kidneys and liver, where it binds to other essential minerals and vitamins, so preventing their utilisation. In their study on mineral status in new babies, Bryce-Smith and Ward also found that cadmium levels are higher in the placentae of those stillborn or born with spina bifida. Greater accumulation of cadmium is also associated with low birth-weight and small head circumference (therefore reduced brain size). And it reduces fertility in both men and women.

Our main sources of cadmium are from cigarette smoke (direct or passive – according to the Health Education Authority, only 15 per cent of the smoke from a cigarette is inhaled by the smoker – the rest goes into the air and is inhaled by those close by) and refined grains found in processed foods. Cadmium is also widely used by the manufacturing industries and has even been found in shellfish from polluted waters. See chapter 4 for more on smoking.

Aluminium: a brain toxin

In areas where there are high levels of aluminium in the water, studies have shown that there is a 50 per cent greater risk of developing Alzheimer's.[41] Like many toxic metals, aluminium binds to essential vitamins and minerals, so seriously compromises nutritional status. Although we know it interferes with brain function and memory, aluminium has also been linked to kidney problems in babies and behavioural problems and autism in children.[42] The main sources of aluminium are antacids, antiperspirants and food additives. Water can also be contaminated, and using aluminium cookware and eating foil-wrapped foods can increase exposure.

Analysing your mineral status

Now we've identified the many potential toxins in the environment, you may be wondering to what extent you're affected. The only way to really find out is to have a hair mineral analysis. This method is the most reliable indicator of what and how much toxic metal has accumulated in your body tissue (your hair being a perfect example, unless it's dyed or permed). This test can also identify deficiencies in minerals essential for fertility and pregnancy such as zinc. A hair mineral analysis is relatively inexpensive and quick to do, but you'll need to see a nutritional therapist to arrange one (see the Resources section for details). Testing both yourself and your partner would normally be included in any preconception consultation.

If high levels of toxic metals are detected, then it's possible with the right diet and supplements to detoxify them and bring your mineral status back into a healthy balance.

Detoxify your body

The most effective way to reduce levels of toxic pollutants in your body is to carefully balance your nutrition. Eating a wholefood, nutrient-rich diet such as the Better Pregnancy Diet (outlined in Part Two) is the best place to start. However, there are specific foods that you can incorporate into your diet to speed up the detoxification process.

- Calcium and phosphorus are antagonistic to lead. They are found in seeds, nuts, green leafy vegetables and dairy produce (but choose organic).

- Alginic acid is also a lead antagonist. It is found in seaweed (provided it comes from unpolluted waters). If seaweed sounds unappetising, try nori. This comes in dried sheets (from good supermarkets or healthfood shops), which can be crisped by heating without oil in a very hot pan for less than ten seconds, and used as a crunchy garnish for soups and salads.

- Pectin helps remove lead too. It is found in apple pips, bananas, citrus fruit and carrots.

- Sulphur-containing amino acids, which are found in garlic, onions and eggs, help protect against mercury, cadmium and lead.

Supplements against pollution

If you find or suspect you have high levels of a particular toxic metal, for example because you are/were a smoker, live in busy city or a heavy farming area where levels of pesticides are higher, have a mouth full of dental fillings, have eaten tuna every day for years or have always used aluminium cookware, you can supplement a healthy diet with additional nutrients. Where body levels of toxins are too high, diet alone cannot supply nutritional antagonists in doses high enough to be effective. Several research projects have shown, however, that certain nutrients are very effective in supplement form.

- Vitamin C is an 'all rounder', which escorts lead and cadmium out of the body.

- Calcium is effective against lead, cadmium and aluminium.

- Zinc acts against lead and cadmium.

- Selenium is antagonistic to mercury and, to a lesser extent, arsenic and cadmium.

- Pectin, alginic acid and phosphorus are also detoxifying and can be useful as supplements.

- Magnesium and B6 are useful for detoxifying aluminium.

Protect yourself from pollution

Toxic minerals are in the air, the soil and our food. Over the past 100 years, their levels have risen sharply and in many cases they overload the body's capacity to eliminate them. Here's what to do to keep your exposure to the minimum.

- Avoid busy roads and smoky atmospheres where possible.

- Remove outer leaves of vegetables and thoroughly wash all fresh produce in a vinegar solution (just add a dessertspoon of vinegar to a bowl of water) to remove pollutants.

- Limit your intake of tuna or non-organic farmed salmon to no more than once a week, if at all, and aim to eat fish from less polluted waters (i.e. Arctic salmon, haddock, cod and sole).

- Avoid copper and aluminium cookware and don't wrap food in aluminium foil (or, if you do, put a layer of greaseproof paper in between foil and food).

- Avoid canned goods, which may be contaminated with aluminium or lead.

- Cut down on alcohol (and avoid it before and during pregnancy), which increases lead and cadmium absorption.

- Avoid antacids, which can contain aluminium salts.

- Avoid refined foods, which lack toxin-fighting nutrients.

- Check if your water pipes are made of lead or copper. If so don't use a water softener. Soft water dissolves lead more easily; do not drink or cook with hot tap water; use a water filter or drink distilled or spring water.

- Take a good antioxidant supplement (see the Resources section for suppliers).

Why organic is ideal

More than 25 million tonnes of pesticides are applied to conventional crops each year in the UK and residues are found on nearly half of all fruit and vegetables tested and one in three of all foods. Multiple residues of up to seven different compounds are not uncommon on many foods, and although it's not yet fully known what the combined effect of multiple compounds might be, some research suggests they could be hundreds of times more toxic than the same compounds individually.

As well as being particularly damaging to a developing foetus and implicated in miscarriages, researchers have linked pesticide levels in patients' bloodstreams with symptoms such as headaches, tremor, lack of energy, depression, anxiety, poor memory, dermatitis, convulsions, nausea, indigestion and diarrhoea. Many pesticides are known or suspected hormone disrupters and the US Environmental Protection Agency ranks pesticide residues among the top three environmental cancer risks.

Nearly all of the 447 pesticides allowed in non-organic farming are prohibited in organic farming and the four that are allowed are generally used on a non-routine basis only following authorisation from the certifying body when all other pest control methods have failed. They are generally simpler substances than those used in non-organic agriculture, tending to degrade more quickly in the environment, and therefore residues are rarely found on organic food.

In addition to fewer pesticides, fewer food additives are permitted in organic processing, genetic modification is completely prohibited and there is no record of any case of BSE, suspected of being linked to new variant CJD (mad cow disease) in humans, in any animal born and reared organically.

Organic food also contains more nutrients. Artificial fertilisers produce lush growth that swells fruit and vegetables with more water – good news for the farmer (higher yields) but not so good for the consumer (less carrot in your carrot and the nutrients in fruit and vegetables are more diluted). According to official data from the old MAFF (now Defra) and the Royal Society of Chemistry, nutrient levels in fruit and vegetables are lower now than they were sixty years ago. Trace minerals in vegetables have fallen by up to 76 per cent. Yet studies comparing the nutrient contents of organic and non-organic fruit and vegetables reveal a strong trend towards higher levels of nutrients in organic produce. Of twenty-seven comparisons of the mineral and vitamin C contents of organic and non-organic crops, fourteen showed higher levels in organic produce while just one favoured non-organic.[43]

So can organic food, with fewer toxins and more nutrients, make a difference to your health? Observations, experience and clinical evidence from organisations such as Foresight (the preconceptual care charity) and the Nutritional Cancer Therapy Trust suggest that it can, but it's very difficult to do any controlled studies with people because of the many other confounding factors, such as genes and lifestyle. Controlled animal feeding trials are interesting, and the evidence here is clear – animals fed organically produced feed have better health in terms of growth, reproductive health and recovery from illness than those fed on non-organic feed, even over successive generations.

Many supermarkets now stock organic produce and organic box delivery schemes are spreading in number throughout the UK. There are also a number of online organic ordering services. See the Resources section for more details.

In summary, to safeguard yourself against pollutants and anti-nutrients:

- **Eat** a nutrient-rich wholefood diet to provide good levels of all the vitamins and minerals that help prevent toxins such as lead, cadmium, aluminum and mercury accumulating. Such a diet is outlined in the Better Pregnancy Diet in Part Two.

- **Take** a good antioxidant supplement, plus extra vitamin C and a multivitamin providing reasonable levels of calcium, magnesium, zinc, selenium and B6.

- **Check** your home for lead pipes or paint, drink filtered or bottled water and don't use copper or aluminium cookware.

- **If** you are concerned about your exposure to pollutants, have a hair mineral analysis to check for toxicity.

- **Eat** organic food wherever possible – in descending order, the priority is: meat and dairy products, grains, root vegetables, vegetables and fruit you cannot peel or remove the outer leaves from, vegetables and fruit you can.

&

CHAPTER FOUR

Drinking, Smoking and Passive Smoking: How Much is Safe?

IF YOU SMOKE you are no doubt aware that this isn't ideal if you're pregnant, but perhaps hope you can get away with cutting right back. If you drink alcohol you may also wonder whether there's any harm in having the odd tipple. The reason why this is such a controversial issue is that both drinking alcohol and smoking are associated with increased risk of birth defects, increased risk of miscarriage – yet we like doing them!

The fact is that, today, more than ever before, miscarriage is the greatest threat to any pregnancy. According to the Miscarriage Association, more than one in five pregnancies ends in miscarriage – that's at least 250,000 babies in the UK each year. Even this figure is likely to be conservative since early miscarriages are often not reported and may even go unnoticed.[44]

Experts believe that miscarriage is the most sensitive of all indications that a woman or her partner are exposed to environmental hazards. Researchers from Columbia University in New York decided to investigate the risk factors associated with miscarriage in 2,802 New York women. They found that rates of miscarriage increased in line with consumption of cigarettes and alcohol. A drinker and smoker was four times more likely to have a miscarriage. Those who didn't smoke but had a drink every day still had a risk more than two-and-half times higher than those who abstained.

Miscarriage: the alcohol connection

Certainly the most widespread poison for an unborn child is alcohol. Drinking just five glasses of wine a week can more than treble your chances of miscarriage, according to a seven-year study at Denmark's Arhus University. Of nearly 25,000 women studied, those who drank five or more units of alcohol a week were almost four times more likely to lose their baby in the early stages of pregnancy. Scientists believe alcohol can cause chromosomal defects in the sperm or egg prior to conception, or trigger the release of toxic chemicals during pregnancy that can cause the death of an unborn baby.

Numerous other studies highlight the damaging effects of even smaller quantities of alcohol during pregnancy. But this knowledge is nothing new. More than 3,000 years ago, the Bible (Judges: 13) records a messenger from God warning Samson's mother: 'You are going to conceive and have a son. Now see to it that you drink no wine or other fermented drink.' In the ancient cities of Carthage and Sparta, newly-weds were banned from drinking alcohol to prevent 'conception during intoxication'. Then in response to health concerns arising from Britain's 'gin epidemic' in the 1720s, the Royal College of Physicians reported to Parliament that parental drinking was a cause of 'weak, feeble and distempered children'.

But it wasn't until 1967 that a team of French doctors first studied and described in scientific terms a group of children affected by maternal alcohol abuse.[45] And as these ideas usually take some time to filter into the mainstream, it took a further fourteen years for a landmark report in the *International Journal of Environmental Studies* actually to identify that 'alcohol is the third most common environmental cause of difficulties in the development of an unborn child.[46] So let's examine the evidence.

How your baby is affected by alcohol

Miscarriage may be nature's way of terminating a pregnancy that is destined to go wrong, but many babies are nevertheless born suffering from the effects of maternal alcohol consumption. In the extreme, the signs and symptoms are known as foetal alcohol syndrome (FAS). According to a report in the *New Scientist*, 'Its main signs are low birth-weight and mild facial deformity. The flattened midface, often with a thin upper lip, is connected to a short nose with little nostril flare. The eyelid openings are short, the ears often misshapen, and the lower jaw long. Many affected babies also have heart murmurs, persistent ear infections leading to deafness, droopy eyelids, squint, congenital hip dislocations, and fingers and toes that may be short, partly fused, angled, lacking in flexion, and with small nails.'[47] These are the most common physical abnormalities seen in children whose mothers consumed too much alcohol during pregnancy.

But alcohol affects mental development and behaviour too. Babies born with FAS are often hyperactive, jittery and have difficulty sleeping – just like an adult withdrawing from alcohol.[48] However, a baby doesn't have to have any obvious physical signs to be mentally defected by alcohol. While FAS is now recognised as the leading known case of mental retardation – surpassing Down's syndrome and spina bifida[49] – even small quantities of drink can affect a baby's brain development and function. Babies exposed to alcohol in the womb have smaller brains with fewer and differently distributed brain cells, and this causes varying degrees of mental deficiency – from mild behavioural problems to obvious mental handicap.[50] Low birth-weight and congenital abnormalities have also been linked to the negative effects of alcohol, and studies show there is also twice the risk of abnormalities.[51]

How much is too much?

While the social norm may be a few glasses of wine here and there, Dr Woollam, a consultant to the World Health Organisation who has undertaken thirty years of research into environmental hazards including thalidomide, says: 'No alcohol during pregnancy is the only safe limit.' His views are backed up by a study from Columbia University that showed that even the consumption of a single drink every other day increased the risk of miscarriage.

The UK Department of Health, in 2007, changed its advice for pregnant women and recommended that they abstain completely – a view we've held for many years. This view is supported by scientists at Queen's University in Belfast. Researchers there produced a study showing that even a tiny amount of alcohol (four glasses of wine a week) can affect an unborn baby's brain and nervous system, and warned that women who drink during pregnancy will give birth to children with shorter attention spans, who find it harder to do well at school.

Many environmental hazards, including alcohol, are at their most dangerous at the very early stages of pregnancy, when your baby's rate of development is at its highest. So alcohol really needs to be avoided from the time you and your partner start trying to get pregnant, not just when you discover you are. Ideally, it should also be limited for a period prior to preconception if you want to ensure your egg and your partner's sperm are of optimal quality. In the same way as if you were planting a tree, the quality of the seeds are just as important as the actual nurturing and growing. For more on this, read chapter 1.

Once pregnant, although the first twenty weeks are deemed the most critical stage during which alcohol should be avoided, there is clear evidence to show it can cause damage at any time. Dr Ann Streissguth, who was one of the first doctors to identify the characteristics of FAS, says that 'Experiments on animals demonstrate that babies exposed to alcohol only in the later stages of pregnancy are still susceptible to behavioural problems.'[52] And while it had been hoped that children would grow out of these physical and mental defects, it is now clear that they don't. In a follow-up study on ten FAS children by Dr Streissguth, two are dead, and the rest are physically and mentally impaired.

So although it may be tough, save the champagne until after the birth, and even then don't have too much if you are breast feeding!

The effects of smoking on the unborn child – by either parent

Cyanide, carbon monoxide, lead, cadmium and ammonia are all deadly substances, yet these – plus some 600 further chemicals that give off thousands of toxic compounds once lit – are added to tobacco to make cigarettes. Despite the 500 or so scientific papers published each year that highlight the dangers of smoking, most smokers start young, when cancer, heart disease and the other serious health risks that a love affair with tobacco inevitably brings, seem too far away to be tangible. Yet to unborn children, exposure to smoke in their first nine months of life (and even before, when sperm and eggs are being produced or matured in the parents) can reduce growth, cause malformations, impair mental development and increase their risk of death.

Despite its 'herbal' connotations that suggest it's somehow safer, research into cannabis shows similar toxic side effects to tobacco. In animals, its consumption has been linked to stillbirths and malformations.[53] Impaired mental functioning, reduced IQ and hyperactivity have been reported in children born to cannabis-smoking parents, and other research has found that regular cannabis consumption can reduce sperm count and cause impotence in men.[54]

Although smoking anything while pregnant has thankfully become a social taboo, many women don't realise that they are pregnant until the first few weeks have passed, so unwittingly expose their unborn child to tobacco toxins at a crucial time of its development. As smoking is also highly addictive, it may then take more time before they are able to kick the habit completely. And considering that the most regular and heaviest smokers are women and men of childbearing age, the chances are if you're a smoker, your partner is one too. So while you're both reducing your likelihood of conceiving in the first place, you're also damaging the raw materials that will make a baby – the egg and sperm – and this can have a dramatic impact on your child's future health.

Smoking and malformations in babies

Studies have found that babies born to parents who smoke are more likely to suffer malformations – in particular, cleft palates, hare lips, deafness and squints. The reason is believed to be because smoking damages the way cells replicate and also interferes with protein synthesis (i.e. building new cells), both vital when building a new human being.[55] As these are at their most rapid in the first few weeks following conception, smoking in the early stages of pregnancy is even more damaging.

Babies exposed to cigarette smoke in the womb are also found to have increased heart rates, and research has found that children born to mothers who smoke have a higher instance of heart defects compared with those born to non-smoking mothers.[56]

Even if you don't smoke, if your partner does, your risk for having a baby with birth defects still increases by two-and-half times. Research has found that the mutagenic compounds of tobacco damage the chromosomes (the cells that unite at conception to make a baby) of sperm.[57] As it takes about four months to produce sperm (a month or so more than the time taken to mature an egg), encouraging your partner to stop smoking long before you plan to try for a baby is therefore crucial.

Smoking and growth rate

About 54,000 babies are born prematurely or with a low birth-weight every year in the UK. While there can be many reasons for this, the main factor is believed to be maternal smoking during pregnancy.[58]

The effect on birth size is caused by the ability of cigarette smoke to slow down the rate of growth of your baby. It does this by reducing oxygen and decreasing blood flow to your womb, which means the baby receives fewer nutrients. Cadmium (a highly toxic metal) from cigarette smoke also interferes with the body's ability to store and use the essential mineral zinc, which is vital, among other things, for an unborn baby's growth. These factors in combination reduce the size and weight of a baby when it's born. Birth-weight is so key because it is a strong predictor of health in later life (see page 138). The average reported weight reduction in babies born to smokers can fluctuate between 4.2oz (120g) and 15oz (430g) or more, depending on how many cigarettes are smoked.[59]

Cigarette smoke also damages DNA, our blueprint for survival. This in turn has far more serious consequences for mental and physical development, as well as increasing the risk of having a premature baby.[60] The risk of miscarriage is also greater – by as much as 27 per cent compared to non-smokers.[61]

While the toxic effect of cigarettes is what undoubtedly causes so much damage, the power of good nutrition is such that it appears to be able to counter some of the effects. In a study in which women were divided according to expected birth-weight of offspring, then either given multivitamin supplements or not, there was a significant difference in weight of baby between those who smoked more than ten cigarettes a day and were supplemented, and those who smoked and were not. The supplementation appeared to offer some protection against the risk of low birth-weight.[62]

Smoking and intelligence

The effects of maternal smoking can be seen many years later in the child. A massive survey at Pennsylvania State University involving 9,024 cases looked at differences between children who were born to the same mothers, but where the mother only smoked during one of the pregnancies. Those children who were born following a smoking pregnancy were more likely to be hyperactive, have shorter attention spans and score lower on spelling and reading tests than their siblings.[63]

Antisocial behaviour is also more common in children born to smokers. A study in the early 1990s found a 10.3 per cent incidence of delinquency by the age of twenty-two among sons born to mothers who smoked during pregnancy, compared to 4.6 per cent in sons of non-smokers.[64]

Smoking and illness in children

An important concept in nutrition today is that of 'organ reserve'. It's like being born with £100 in the bank. If an organ comes under pressure, that bank reserve drops. Eventually the reserve will run out and the organ will malfunction. For example, those with weak immune systems become more susceptible to infections, or those with poor hormone and nerve balance succumb to the ravages of stress. Children born to mothers who smoke appear to have an overall poor organ reserve, as illustrated by their greater susceptibility to illness. Dr Paula Rantakallio, a Finnish researcher, compared the health of children of smokers compared to non-smokers and found a 43 per cent increase in illnesses among the smokers' children. These included more respiratory infections, nervous system and sense disorders, blood disorders, bladder and kidney problems and more skin disorders.[65]

How to stop smoking

By now you have probably got the message that smoking before and during pregnancy is very bad news. But what can you do to stop? For the hardened smoker, simply throwing your cigarettes in the bin and going cold turkey is the strategy with the least likelihood of success. You need to support your body through the withdrawal – after all tobacco is more addictive than heroin. The diet outlined in this book will certainly help, as the foods it promotes will balance your blood sugar, which means you're less likely to suffer from the energy lows that make you crave cigarettes. There are also tried and tested habit-breaking techniques and specific supplements you can take. See www.how2quit.co.uk or read *How to Quit Without Feeling S**t* (Piatkus).

Don't forget to encourage your partner to quit if he's a smoker too. According to the Health Education Authority, only 15 per cent of the smoke from a cigarette is inhaled by the smoker – the rest goes into the air and is inhaled by those close by (i.e. you, and after birth, your baby!).

In summary:

- **Avoid** any alcohol – ideally for at least four months before conception (both you and your partner) and then throughout your pregnancy.

- **Seek** help to give up smoking, encourage your partner to do the same, and don't expose yourself to passive smoking – again, ideally four months before conception and throughout your pregnancy.

CHAPTER FIVE

How to Virtually Eradicate the Risk of Birth Defects

N O ONE LIKES to think about the possibility of having a baby with some kind of defect. Yet, according to Foresight, one in every seventeen babies born today in the UK will have some form of mental or physical abnormality. As we've seen in chapter 4, many pregnancies also end in miscarriage. Although prospective parents think 'it will never happen to me', these statistics are just too high to ignore. That's why it's crucial to understand more about how birth defects occur and what can be done to minimise the risk of anything going wrong with your baby. If you take the right steps now you can massively increase the odds in your favour of having a super-healthy baby.

Your nutritional status at the actual time of conception is the most important factor in the growth of your baby.[66] A poor diet can slow down the rapid growth phase that takes place in the first six weeks of pregnancy, when the cells of your developing baby divide more frequently. Cell division is like doubling numbers – 2, 4, 8, 16, 32, 64, 128 and so on. Leave out one and the reduction in the total number of cells at birth can be appreciable. It has been calculated that the effects of a cell not doubling in early pregnancy can be the difference between a 7lb 11oz (3.5kg) baby and a 5lb 8oz (2.5kg) baby. The other reason this is so key is that low birth-weight babies (defined as 5lb 8oz/2.5kg and under) are at greater risk of abnormalities – neurological defects, for example, are more than three times more common in this group than in babies of optimal weight (between 7lb 11oz and 8lb 13oz/3.5 to 4kg).[67]

Given that most women don't even discover that they are pregnant until several weeks after conceiving, optimum nutrition should ideally start preconceptually to mimimise the risk of birth defects. Diet is obviously key, but research has also shown that taking a multivitamin and mineral supplement prior to conceiving can reduce not only the rate of neural tube defects (e.g. spina bifida) but also other birth abnormalities.[68]

This is because a mother's deficiency in any essential nutrient can cause birth defects and developmental problems in her growing baby. In this section, we've selected the key vitamins and minerals that have been identified by research as having the most significant impact. However, beware supplementing these in isolation as too much of one nutrient that's not balanced with others can also create problems. The best way to protect your baby against birth defects is to eat a healthy diet supplemented with a balanced range of extra nutrients. The Better Pregnancy Diet and Supplement Plan in Part Two provides the ideal programme both during pregnancy and before while you are preparing to conceive. As drinking and smoking before and during pregnancy also contribute to birth defects, eliminating these is also wise. For more on this, read chapter 4.

Prevent spina bifida with folic acid

The importance of folic acid in pregnancy was first recognised in 1970, when Dr Richard Smithells reported a link between insufficient folate (the form of folic acid found in plants) and spina bifida, a congenital defect in which the spinal column is imperfectly closed at birth, often resulting in permanently disabling neurological disorders. It took twenty years for Dr Smithells's work to be taken seriously and then, in 1992, for the first time ever, the US and UK governments recommended a nutritional supplement, saying that women of childbearing age should take 400mcg of folic acid daily, as this amount is not easily achieved by diet alone. This is the first crack ever to appear in the conventional (and, as we see it, false) medical belief that 'as long as you eat a well-balanced diet, you get all the nutrients you need'.

In 1998, the US government went one step further when it introduced mandatory fortification of bread and pasta with folic acid. Spina bifida and other neural tube defects (NTDs) have since declined by almost 20 per cent. The UK government has since followed suit. However, while supplementing folic acid on its own does reduce NTDs, among the elderly those low in vitamin B12 appear to have worsening memory as a result. Also, there is some evidence that, in those with pre-cancerous polyps, folic acid can increase colorectal cancer. It is always better to have all the B vitamins – not just one.

Folic acid belongs to the B vitamin family, which play a crucial role in cell division in a developing embryo and foetus. This includes neural tubes, which develop in the first twenty-eight days of pregnancy, often before a woman even realises she is pregnant.

Getting an adequate supply of folic acid both reduces the risk of birth defects and miscarriages[69] and prevents premature birth and low birth-weight.[70] The best dietary sources include green leafy vegetables, wholegrains (such as brown rice, rye or wholemeal bread), organ meats, milk and salmon. But sunlight, heat or an acid environment easily destroy it, so unless we eat very fresh and/or raw food, it's hard to get sufficient quantities. The folate form of folic acid is also thought to be manufactured by the 'friendly' bacteria in our intestinal tract. But overuse of antibiotics can destroy these bacteria, and this can also contribute to a deficiency. Folic acid is the form of folate used in vitamin supplements and has been proven to be up to twice as effective as the equivalent in food.[71]

Although the Department of Health recommends a daily intake of 400mcg for all young women (we recommend 600mcg before and during pregnancy), the average daily intake in Britain is less than 200mcg. During pregnancy, your baby draws on your folic acid stores for its own growth, but a deficiency may not cause any obvious signs in you. So to be sure you're getting enough, take a supplement that also gives you a good balance of all the other essential vitamins and minerals (see chapter 12 for details about supplements). According to Dr Carl Pfeiffer, an American nutritional biochemist, 'Many women with histories of abortion and miscarriage have been able to complete successful childbirth subsequent to folic acid supplementation.'

Minerals that make healthy babies

Another key nutrient involved in preventing birth abnormalities is manganese. In a study from Istanbul, the concentration of manganese in human hair was measured in mothers and babies. Babies who were born with congenital malformations were significantly lower in hair manganese, as were their mothers. This suggests that manganese deficiency may be another cause for birth abnormalities.[72]

Low zinc can also have a negative effect on pregnancy. Research shows that pregnant animals deficient in this crucial mineral are more prone to miscarriage and stillbirth or giving birth to young with a range of defects such as brain malformations, impaired immune systems, cleft palettes and genitourinary abnormalities. In a study at the University of Surrey, the zinc status of women who had had a healthy pregnancy with a healthy baby at the end of it was significantly higher than that of women who'd experienced problems (including having babies with birth defects). As your zinc levels can decrease by as much as 30 per cent during pregnancy (undoubtedly due to the huge demands of building a new human being), ensuring you're getting enough prior to and throughout pregnancy is essential.

Food sources and supplements of all these key minerals are discussed in more detail in chapters 10, 11 and 12.

Vitamin A: is caution needed?

You may have heard that it's dangerous to take vitamin A when you're pregnant, but the message is different depending on where you live. Some British pregnancy supplement manufacturers deliberately leave it out of their formulas. Yet the United Nations Educational, Scientific and Cultural Organisation (UNESCO) campaigns for funding to give vitamin A to pregnant mothers in developing countries to stop their babies being born blind. And if you are pregnant in the US, it's recommended you take 5,000IUs a day; 10,000IUs in parts of Australia.

Why so much variation? The concerns over too much vitamin A came about for two reasons. Firstly, there is a case of one woman eating vast quantities of liver – one of the richest sources of vitamin A – during her pregnancy, who gave birth to a malformed baby. And secondly, the acne medication Roaccutane uses a synthetic form of vitamin A (isotretinoin) that's been found to be highly toxic to a developing baby. It's so toxic that women must first sign a termination consent before they can be prescribed it to be sure they won't continue with a pregnancy if they conceive during treatment.

However, vitamin A is essential in pregnancy for the healthy development of your baby's eyes, heart and reproductive system, and studies have shown that women who supplement their diets with multivitamins including vitamin A have a lower incidence of birth defects. So it's key to get the right amount but not too much. As there are two kinds of vitamin A – retinol, which is derived from animal sources such as liver and cod liver oil, and betacarotene from vegetables such as carrots and sweet potatoes – this can be confusing. But it's retinol rather than betacarotene that has the potential to be toxic at high levels, so it's unwise for women of childbearing age to supplement any more than 10,000IUs daily unless directed by their doctor or nutritional therapist. As cod liver oil is also a rich source of retinol, check the label for exact quantities if you're taking this – a high-strength formula rarely supplies more than 2,640IUs (800mcg) of retinol, so in practical terms, take no more than four cod liver oil capsules a day just before and during pregnancy.

Reducing the risk of Down's syndrome

Down's syndrome is a chromosomal abnormality caused by fertilisation with a defective egg or sperm. It is more common in babies born to older parents because they have had more exposure to damaging pollutants and the ravages of an unhealthy lifestyle (stress, alcohol, poor diet, etc.). In women, the quality of your eggs also decreases as you get older, which increases the chances of having a baby with Down's. But whatever your age or the age of your partner, you can reduce the risk by minimising all that damages your body (read chapters 3 and 4) and maximising all that improves your health (all the advice contained in this book!). Having high levels of a naturally occurring substance called homocysteine can also increase your chances of having a Down's baby. Testing for and reducing this is discussed in chapter 6.

Even in children born with Down's, studies have shown that optimum nutrition can boost IQ between 10 and 25 points.[73] This has meant that children previously classed as having severe learning difficulties were able to switch to normal schooling. For more on this, read *Optimum Nutrition for the Mind* (see Resources).

The role of nutrition in brain development

The brain is the most complicated part of any human being and also the most vulnerable. This mere 3lb (1,300g) of delicate hardware uses up almost half the energy we make from food while we are resting (and up to a third while we are active). In a growing foetus, nerve cells in the brain called neurons are rapidly made and by week twenty, your unborn child has as many neurons as you do. Then the wiring begins. Each neuron must interconnect with other neurons by sending out branches. This process is called arborisation. Each neuron connects up with approximately 10,000 other neurons, forming a remarkably complex and integral web. This is the centre of our intelligence. The process of arborisation still remains a mystery to scientists. Involving both the genetic instructions contained in DNA and feedback through the senses, a newborn baby rapidly develops an intelligence far beyond that of any other living animal.

Arborisation happens towards the end of pregnancy and continues throughout childhood, especially in the early stages of your baby's life. It is assumed, although it is impossible to test for obvious moral and ethical reasons, that nutrition plays a major role in brain development. The mineral zinc, for example, promotes DNA production, and zinc antagonists like lead and cadmium are known, from research, to stunt arborisation by up to 10 per cent in animals.

What we do know about nutrition and brain development is that in small-for-dates babies there are definite signs of mental retardation, manifesting as poor coordination and slow reaction to stimuli.[74] A survey of brain-damaged patients in Finland revealed that 'a remarkably large number of cases have primary cerebral maldevelopment suggesting a pre-natal origin'.[75] The size of head circumference at birth is therefore of primary importance.

More tenuous is the connection between low birth-weight or poor physical growth and intelligence. However, it does appear even here that despite different environments for learning, the intelligence of a child at age six is more likely to be high if birth-weight was high.

The drugs to avoid before and during pregnancy

Very few, if any, drugs are considered safe during pregnancy. Figures from animal research show that 70 per cent of drugs that are dangerous to humans pass tests on primates, and the number that pass rodent tests may be greater still. What's more, most drugs are never tested in clinical trials on pregnant women for obvious ethical reasons. Therefore, it is often not known how the unborn child may react.

Drugs are often low in molecular weight, which means they can pass easily through the placenta into the foetus. The thalidomide disaster debunked once and for all the idea that the placenta protects the foetus from drugs taken by the mother. However, most people put drugs like this in a totally different category from sleeping pills, painkillers or tranquillisers. Although these common drugs do not cause toxic disasters as witnessed by thalidomide, they are still toxic substances that the unborn child is not designed to cope with and they should be avoided where possible.

But it's not just drugs taken during pregnancy. According to

Foresight, the pre-conceptual care charity, women who take medicinal drugs in the three weeks prior to conception have been found to have a higher risk of chromosomal abnormalities in their developing babies.

Are painkillers safe?

Aspirin belongs to a family of medicines called 'non-steroidal anti-inflammatory drugs' (NSAIDs), of which ibuprofen is another member. Many women are prescribed aspirin by their doctor to reduce the risk of miscarriage or pre-eclampsia (a condition where blood pressure becomes dangerously high, causing risk to both mother and baby). Research claims that women taking low doses are less likely to have a stillbirth or to develop pre-eclampsia. Yet more recent research claims that women who take NSAIDs are 80 per cent more likely to have a miscarriage, with the most danger occurring in the early stages of pregnancy.[76] An earlier study also found that children born to mothers who took aspirin in the first half of pregnancy had significantly lower IQs and reduced ability to concentrate.[77]

Our advice, therefore, is to address the source of any pain for which you may need to take regular painkillers before you get pregnant by visiting your doctor or nutritional consultant. If pre-eclampsia is a risk, follow a nutritional strategy to reduce it (see page 135). Beware, too, paracetamol. Often considered a 'safer' painkilling option, it has been linked to cell mutations in both animals and humans.[78]

Even if you're 'drug' free, any medications your partner takes can affect your baby when it's conceived. The common morphine-derivative codeine, for example, can be carried by sperm into the female genital tract and lead to congenital malformations.[79]

The dangers of tranquillisers and sleeping tablets

Benzodiazepines, often prescribed as tranquillisers, can disturb the brain and nervous system in the early stages of pregnancy,[80] which can cause visible malformations and mental disorders in babies who've been exposed. Anti-depressants also pose a danger – babies born to women taking Prozac have an increased risk of minor abnormalities.[81]

Drugs that affect the brain such as tranquillisers, sleeping tablets and alcohol also affect the secretion of hormones that control the menstrual cycle and sustain pregnancy.[82] After ovulation, the follicle from which an ovum is released becomes a supporting structure called a corpus luteum, and this produces progesterone and oestrogen to maintain a pregnancy for the first eight weeks. However, if drugs interfere with the hormones that stimulate the follicle to develop (called gonadatrophic hormones), then it cannot go on to produce sufficient progesterone and oestrogen and leads to what is called a 'blighted ovum' that miscarries.

Reducing the toxicity of drugs with nutrients

Even if a drug is deemed 'safe', the synergistic effect of two or more drugs together (and this could include coffee, alcohol, cigarettes or painkillers, for example) can create a highly adverse reaction, especially in a developing baby whose immune system is not yet formed. Drugs also interact with nutrients. Alcohol, for example, increases excretion of B vitamins (of which folic acid is one), zinc and magnesium – all essential for the development of a defect-free, healthy baby.

So, if you have a condition that needs regular medication, discuss the best way to manage treatment before and during your pregnancy with your doctor. Or seek alternative solutions. Nutritional therapy can help to successfully treat pain, inflammation, stress, insomnia and depression, among others, without the need for drugs. Other complementary therapies such as homoeopathy or herbalism can also provide long-term solutions that won't harm your baby.

However, it is inevitable that some pregnant women may need to be prescribed a drug during pregnancy. If this happens to you, the potential danger can be reduced by ensuring nutrition is optimum. Even drugs like thalidomide were found to become more toxic if vitamin deficiency existed. Deficiencies of vitamins A, B2, pantothenic acid (B5), folic acid, B12 and E all increased the risk of birth defects with thalidomide. In the words of the Swiss physician Paracelsus, 'Only the dose makes the poison,' and vitamin deficiency effectively lowers the dose that can be tolerated without ill effect.

Protecting your baby's future health

Babies born to mothers who have poor nutrition before and during pregnancy – even if they appear perfectly healthy at birth – are more likely to develop health problems later in life. For example, there is a link with a greater risk of heart disease.[83] Other research has shown that if a woman isn't adequately nourished before conceiving, while she may give birth to a normal weight baby, that child's own baby is at greater risk of being of low birth-weight (see page 138).

So, making sure you get the best possible diet, backed up with the right balance of nutrients and compromised by as few pollutants as possible, is crucial not only for the growing a defect-free baby while you're pregnant, but for that baby's future health after birth and throughout its life.

In summary, to protect your unborn baby from developing birth defects:

- **Plan** your pregnancy to give you and your partner time to become optimally nourished and reduce your exposure to harmful sub-stances such as alcohol, tobacco and drugs (both recreational and pharmaceutical) before you conceive.

- **Start** taking a multivitamin and mineral supplement that provides 600mg of folic acid plus 10mg of zinc and 2mg of manganese (see also chapter 12 for other suggested nutrient levels).

- **Ensure** you get enough vitamin A but don't exceed 10,000IU of the retinol form.

- **If** you have to take a drug of any sort, ensure your body is opti-mally nourished to minimise any toxic side effects.

∾

CHAPTER SIX

Your 'H' Score – the Hallmark of a Healthy Pregnancy

Most women know that folic acid is a key nutrient to take both before and during pregnancy. The reason is that folic acid lowers your blood homocysteine level, or H score, and having a high homocysteine is bad news for your baby, contributing to defects such as spina bifida.

But even those who supplement folic acid can still have problems conceiving, repeated miscarriages, premature births or other pregnancy problems, or sometimes bear children with mental or physical defects. Why? Because the only way to guarantee a low H score is to supplement B2, B6, B12, zinc and magnesium, as well as folic acid.

Homocysteine and methylation

The reason why homocysteine is probably the single, most important indicator of a healthy pregnancy is twofold. First, homocysteine is a toxin and damages the placenta if you have too much in the blood. Second, and most important, homocysteine reflects a critical chemical process in the body called 'methylation' and being a 'good methylator' is what allows cells to divide and grow to full bloom.

Methylation is a biochemical process that makes essential substances and breaks down toxic ones in the body – we methylate about one billion times a second. Methylation is responsible not only for ensuring healthy reproductive function, but it also determines our mood, immune function and how quickly we age. However, in around 10 per cent of the population, this process is genetically impaired, while in many others it's not as efficient as it should be due to a low intake of the essential nutrients that aid methylation.

Why methylation is so key for pregnancy

According to Dr Adrian Bird of Edinburgh University, 'One in four gene mutations that cause human disease can be attributed to methyl groups on our genes'. This vital biochemical process is specifically involved with:

- the formation of hormones such as oestrogen, progesterone and insulin

- energy production in every cell

- synthesising and repairing RNA and DNA (i.e. our genetic blueprint), hence all cellular growth

- controlling how genetic material is incorporated in a developing baby

- detoxification (e.g. eliminating heavy metals from mercury to lead)

- mobilising and eliminating fats and cholesterol.

So how do you know if you're a good or a bad methylator? A simple test can measure a protein-like substance called homocysteine, which occurs at the start of the methylation pathway (see chart opposite). Your results come in the form of a numerical score – if you have a low level (below 6), then it shows that you are able to convert homocysteine easily and that your methylation pathway is working efficiently. However, if like many, you have a high level (above 12) and you are not as efficient at converting it, then this substance can cause havoc.

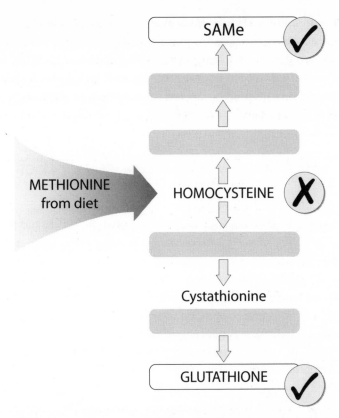

The Homocysteine Pathway: methionine, absorbed from protein in the diet, is converted to homocysteine, which should then be converted to the beneficial substances SAMe or glutathione. However, if key nutrients are lacking, then homocysteine can get stuck and build up, which is harmful.

Research has traditionally linked high homocysteine with cardiovascular disease (strokes, heart attacks, angina, etc.). However, scientists are now finding that it's implicated in more than fifty different diseases and medical conditions including infertility, pregnancy problems and birth defects. So strong is the link between these problems and homocysteine that we strongly recommend that any woman who either intends to get pregnant or has just become pregnant has a homocysteine test as soon as possible.

If your homocysteine level (or H score) is high, you know that you are insufficiently nourished in the nutrients essential for methylation – these are B2, B6, B12, zinc and trimethylglycine (or TMG). In an ideal world, you should not get pregnant until your H score is below 6 because this minimises the risk of problems in pregnancy. Let's examine the evidence.

High homocysteine increases the risk of pregnancy problems

As part of a large-scale study in Norway called the Hordaland Homocysteine Study, investigators measured homocysteine in over 5,800 pre-menopausal Norwegian women between the ages of forty and forty-two. They compared homocysteine levels with the women's previous pregnancy outcomes as recorded by a medical birth registry.[84]

Women with higher homocysteine levels were 32 to 101 per cent more likely to have experienced pregnancy complications such as preeclampsia, premature birth and low birth-weight babies. Birth defects including neural tube defects (such as spina bifida) and clubfoot also occurred more frequently in babies whose mothers had higher levels of homocysteine, a finding that has been confirmed by other research groups.[85]

A separate Dutch study found a similar result and concluded that high homocysteine and/or low folic acid can indicate risk factors for repeated early pregnancy loss. Among women who experienced repeated miscarriages, those with higher homocysteine levels had roughly a three- to fourfold greater risk of suffering further miscarriages.[86] Women who have had early miscarriages are also more likely to have babies born with defects, both of which are more common if your H score is higher.[87]

The good news is that knowing your H score doesn't just predict whether you're at risk. It also provides the answer to reducing that risk – namely, improving your diet (as outlined in the Better Pregnancy Diet in Part Two) and supplementing key nutrients such as extra B vitamins, zinc and TMG, which can be found in single formulas. This is especially key if you are one of the 10 per cent of pre-menopausal women who have a common genetic defect impairing your ability to methylate.

Homocysteine damages the placenta

Having a high homocysteine level not only indicates that you are sub-optimal in certain key nutrients, it also damages a key organ of pregnancy, the placenta. As a result, other essential nutrients, such an important Omega 3 fat called DHA, can't be well enough supplied from mother to baby during pregnancy. Babies born with birth defects consistently have lower DHA levels and high homocysteine levels.[88]

Homocysteine-lowering nutrients

As we've said in chapter 5, folic acid is key to a healthy pregnancy, and supplementing with at least 400mcg a day is well proven to minimise the risk of birth defects. If you find your homocysteine level is high, then higher levels of folic acid will be needed to bring your H score down (see page 62). However, folic acid is not the only nutrient essential for a healthy pregnancy and a healthy H score.

Vitamins B6 and B12 also lower homocysteine and reduce the risk of birth defects and miscarriages. Other essential nutrients include zinc and Omega 3 fats (found in oily fish, flaxseed and nuts), both important in reducing homocysteine and optimising methylation, which as we've seen is the chemical process that transforms one biochemical into another. Zinc is especially important to supplement since the optimal intake of zinc is 20mg during pregnancy, which is a long way short of the average daily intake of 7.6mg.

As well as folic acid, B6, B12 and zinc, vitamin B2, TMG and magnesium are also important nutrients for lowering homocysteine. But how much do you need? Everyone is different. But by measuring your H score, you can see whether or not your current intake is enough. If your score is high, then you need more to bring it down and maintain it below a level of 6.

Getting tested for homocysteine

You can get a homocysteine test done via a nutritional therapist (see the Resources section), or your doctor may do it for you on the NHS. There's also a home test that you can do yourself through Yorktest Laboratories (again, see Resources for contact details).

The average H score is around 10. If you have the genetic defect mentioned earlier, then your score is likely to be much higher. However, no matter what your score, with the right diet (the Better Pregnancy Diet outlined in Part Two) and supplements (see below), it's possible to bring your score down to below 6 in about three months or less.

The supplements are all quite safe to take before and during pregnancy. The ideal protocol is to take them at the levels corresponding to your score for three months, then retest and reduce the amounts to those that correspond to your new score. You ideally want to get your homocysteine below 6 and keep it there before conceiving. If you are already pregnant, you can still follow the programme to bring it down before you give birth.

Nutrient	H Score			
	Below 6 (no risk)	6–9 (low risk)	9–15 (high risk)	Above 15 (very high risk)
Folic acid	200mcg	400mcg	1,200mcg	2,000mcg
B12	10mcg	500mcg	1,000mcg	1,500mcg
B6	25mg	50mg	75mg	100mg
B2	10mg	15mg	20mg	50mg
Zinc	5mg	10mg	15mg	20mg
TMG	500mg	750mg	1.5–3g	3-6g

There's no need to rattle with pills – rather than buying these nutrients separately, many companies produce formulas that combine all or most of them in a few daily tablets. See the Resources section for details.

If you want to find out more about homocysteine, read Patrick's book (co-authored with Dr James Braly), *The Homocysteine Solution* (see Resources).

In summary:

- **Get** your homocysteine tested – ideally before you plan to conceive.

- **Follow** the Better Pregnancy Diet and Supplement Plan, outlined in Part Two.

- **Take** additional supplements at appropriate levels to reduce your H score to below 6 and keep it there.

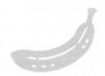

CHAPTER SEVEN

Banish Allergies and Boost Immunity

As YOU EMBARK on creating another life, there is no more crucial time for your health to be optimal. Not only do you want to give your baby the best possible start, but you also want to look and feel the best you can. With so many people now suffering from allergies that cause unpleasant reactions and restrict their diet, identifying any substances that may trigger such a response in you is not only the first step to improving your own health, but also reduces the risk that you will pass on your allergies to your unborn child. This is especially important since researchers believe that allergies can start during pregnancy. Babies who are uncomfortably active in the womb may be trying to tell you they don't like the room service! It could also be the very first sign of food-allergy-induced hyperactivity. So the place to start preventing food allergies in your baby is with yourself.

Boosting your immune system will also help to banish any allergies you currently have and reduce your likelihood of developing further allergies in the future. It will also improve your overall resistance to illness and disease, which is particularly key in pregnancy as some viruses can damage an unborn baby. But even if you only get a cold or two in the nine months you're pregnant, not being able to reach for your usual medication can make the symptoms feel worse.

Understanding allergies

Cases of allergies are increasing and are now thought to affect one in three people. Some people react to airborne substances such as pollen (hayfever), house dust mite or cat fur, others to chemicals in food, household products or environmental toxins. But the most common category of all allergy-provoking substances is the food we eat.

Classic symptoms of food intolerance include:

- Nausea
- Cramps
- Flatulence
- Fatigue
- Throat trouble
- Sweating
- Skin rashes
- Acne and boils
- Migraine
- Apathy and confusion
- Depression
- Anxiety and paranoia

In a survey of 3,300 American adults 43 per cent said they experienced adverse reactions to food.[89] If you experience one or more of the symptoms above on a regular basis, it's highly likely that what you're eating is causing an allergic reaction.

The common definition of an allergy is 'any idiosyncratic reaction where the immune system is clearly involved'. The immune system, which is the body's defence system, has the ability to produce 'markers' for substances it doesn't like. The classic markers are antibodies called IgE. When an offending food (called an 'allergen') is consumed, an IgE antibody reacts and triggers the release of histamine and other chemicals that cause a common allergic reaction – skin rashes, hayfever, rhinitis, sinusitis, asthma and/or eczema. Severe food allergies to shellfish or peanuts, for example, can cause immediate gastrointestinal upsets or swelling in the face or throat. All these reactions are immediate, severe, inflammatory reactions. And it's these types of allergies that get passed from mother to child, and therefore run in families.

However, not all reactions are immediate, nor do they involve the IgE family of antibodies. The emerging view now is that most food allergies and intolerances involve other immune cells, specifically an antibody known as IgG, which behave in a different way. According to allergy specialist Dr James Braly:

> Food allergy is not rare, nor are the effects limited to the air passages, the skin and digestive tract. Most food allergies are delayed reactions, taking anywhere from an hour to three days to show themselves, and are therefore much harder to detect. Delayed food allergy appears to be simply the inability of your digestive tract to prevent large quantities of partially digested and undigested food from entering the bloodstream.

What happens when these foods enter the bloodstream is that an IgG antibody 'tags' them. One or two of these 'tags' probably won't cause much of a problem. But if you're eating a lot of a particular food that causes such a reaction – say wheat or dairy three times a day, for example – then you get a gradual build-up of IgG antibodies. 'It is the sheer weight of numbers that causes a problem,' explains Braly. 'These immune complexes are like litter going round in the bloodstream.'

Other immune cells that act like vacuum cleaners then clean up this litter, but in doing so, the activity can cause unpleasant physical side effects, such as headaches, skin rashes or mood swings.

Obviously, this type of IgG allergy puts your body under stress, and any kind of physical stress needs to be minimised as much as possible when you're planning to conceive and while you're pregnant. Once identified and eliminated, it's possible for your body to 'forget' IgG allergy triggers. But it's thought that if you leave them untreated, IgG allergies can develop into IgE allergies – that is, the more immediate and severe type of allergy. And IgE allergies are the type that can be inherited by your baby.

How to identify and eliminate allergies

Because IgE allergies are usually immediate, most people know they have them. For example if you come out in a rash every time you eat strawberries, then you know that you are allergic to them and will therefore probably avoid them. An exception may be those who are allergic to gluten, a type of protein found in wheat, oats, barley and rye. A gluten allergy can lead to a severe inflammatory condition of the digestive tract called coeliac disease, and where this is untreated (often because some sufferers experience little digestive discomfort), it can cause infertility, recurring miscarriages, premature births and low birth-weight babies.[90] Italian obstetricians have recently found undetected coeliac disease to be so common among women who have problem pregnancies that they are advocating all pregnant women are routinely screened for gluten allergy.

If you suspect you have a gluten intolerance – either because you are suffering with any of the allergy-related health issues mentioned so far, or because you find it hard to maintain weight and have unexplained digestive problems – or you believe you are reacting to any food, it's possible to be tested. While your doctor may be able to arrange an allergy test for the more immediate IgE reaction, the technology commonly used by the NHS is unlikely to identify a slower-reacting IgG allergy (in fact, despite the evidence, many doctors don't acknowledge that IgG allergies exist). There are private laboratories that offer blood tests, which can screen for either IgE or IgG allergies (see the Resources section for details of test providers) and you can arrange to be tested independently or through a nutritional therapist.

The exclusion diet route

Other than laboratory testing, perhaps one of the most accurate ways to discover allergens is to follow an 'exclusion diet'. When you eat certain foods every day, it's often hard to pinpoint which, if any, are contributing to any health problems you may be having. So by following an exclusion diet – that is avoiding suspect foods for a set time period, then reintroducing them one at a time – you can more clearly see which cause a reaction. The most common allergens are wheat, dairy, all gluten grains (i.e. wheat, oats, barley and rye), citrus fruits, eggs, nuts, tea, coffee, chocolate and soya. You can work out your potential suspects by asking yourself four questions:

1. What foods (or drinks) do I suspect that I react badly to?

2. What foods do I eat at least once if not more every day?

3. What foods would I find hardest to give up?

4. Which of these foods are in the list of the top allergens?

A food that fulfils all these criteria is a strong suspect. If there is more than one food (and there usually is), you can choose whether to test them all together or one at a time. However, if the foods on your list are staples in your diet (for example, wheat and dairy) you may want to consult a nutritional therapist who can support you through the process and suggest alternative foods for you to eat to ensure your diet is balanced.

Once you're ready to start the exclusion, eliminate the food or foods on your list completely for fifteen days. It's important that you don't eat even a tiny amount, so do check the contents of the foods you eat carefully. It's best to prepare yourself well by stocking up with your allergen-free foods before starting.

After the fifteen days have passed, you do this simple pulse test:

1. Take your pulse at rest (after five minutes sitting down), for sixty seconds. Your pulse can be found inside the bony protuberance on the thumb side of your wrist. Write down your rate.

2. Eat more than usual of the first (or only) food you've been excluding. Take care to eat only the substance for which you are testing. So, for example, if you're testing wheat, eat a water biscuit rather than a piece of bread that also contains yeast (another potential allergen).

3. Take your pulse after ten, thirty and sixty minutes. Write down your rates for sixty seconds.

4. Keep a record of any symptoms over the next twenty-four hours.

If your pulse rate remains static or only increases a bit (under ten extra beats per minute) and you have no apparent reaction within twenty-four hours, reintroduce this food (in moderation) into your diet, and proceed with the same test for the next food. However, if your pulse does noticeably increase by ten beats or more – which can happen if the food prompts your immune system to mount an allergic reaction – or if you have any noticeable symptoms within twenty-four hours, avoid this substance and wait a further forty-eight hours before testing the next item on your list.

Those foods to which you show a reaction should then be avoided for at least six months – and certainly for the period prior to conception and during pregnancy. (You can later reintroduce them and test again for a reaction.) Most major supermarkets now produce 'free-from' ranges of alternatives to wheat and dairy foods. And healthfood shops stock a range of substitutes to commonly eaten foods. But be sure if you're cutting something out, that you're getting nutrients from other sources. For example, if you eliminate oranges and you'd normally eat one a day, have a couple of kiwi fruit or some berries to ensure you're still getting a good daily dietary source of vitamin C. If dairy is on your elimination list, make sure you eat plenty of green leafy vegetables, seeds and almonds, and take a multivitamin and mineral supplement to boost calcium levels. Ideally, if you do discover food intolerances, you should try to see a nutritional therapist who can devise a workable healthy diet for you.

A special note about dairy

Not everyone who reacts to dairy is doing so because of an allergic response. Some people – particularly those of African and Indian origin – are deficient in the enzyme required to break down milk products in the digestive tract and this, rather than an immune-triggered allergic reaction, causes symptoms such as bloating, digestive discomfort and flatulence. So rather than eliminating these foods from your diet completely, you may find relief by supplementing the digestive enzyme lactase (available from healthfood stores, or see the Resources section for supplement suppliers). However, if this doesn't help, then follow the elimination diet and test for an immune reaction.

How long to avoid allergens?

Just how long allergens have to be avoided is an open-ended question. Foods that invoke an IgE type, immediate and pronounced reaction may need to be avoided for life. The 'memory' of IgE antibodies is long term. By contrast, immune cells that produce IgG antibodies have a half-life of six weeks. That means that there are half as many six weeks later. The 'memory' of these antibodies is short term, and within six months there is unlikely to be any residual 'memory' of reaction to a food that's been avoided. While avoiding for six months or for the duration before and during your pregnancy may be ideal, another option, after a strict three-month avoidance, is to 'rotate' foods so that an IgG sensitive food is only eaten once every four days. This reduces the build-up of allergen-antibody complexes and lessens the chances of symptoms of intolerance.

Reducing your allergic potential

When you realise that the gateway between your body and the outside world is the digestive tract, it becomes obvious that food intolerances, often caused by too much undigested food getting through into the bloodstream, are much more common if you have faulty digestion.

An almost inevitable consequence of problems with digestion and absorption is food allergies and sensitivities. The body's immune system is highly active in the digestive tract and acts like the bouncer at the gateway into your body. If foods arrive at the gate undigested, or if the gate is damaged and inflamed, the chaos that ensues makes it highly likely that there will be some 'arrests' by the immune police. This is, in essence, what most food allergies or sensitivities are all about.

Of course, the real answer to stopping allergies is to heal the digestive tract and eat foods that don't stress or irritate it. However, the fact is that if you've already developed allergies you need to first 'undevelop' them by finding out what foods you are currently allergic to and avoiding them long enough to heal the digestive tract and reprogramme the immune police. The best way to help reduce your allergic potential, once you've removed the offending foods, is to optimise your intake of nutrients that help the digestive tract to heal:

- Essential fats, especially Omega 3, by eating fish (three portions a week) and seeds (two tablespoons of mixed flax, sunflower, sesame and pumpkin a day).

- The amino acid glutamine (which helps repair gut-wall damage), by supplementing a heaped teaspoon (about 5g) of glutamine powder, on an empty stomach twenty minutes before breakfast.

- Digestive enzymes (which help break down your food), by supplementing a digestive enzyme with each meal. This is especially helpful during the first month if your 'allergic' symptoms are digestive.

- Zinc, by ensuring your daily supplement programme contains 15mg. Seeds and fish are also high in zinc.

- Vitamin A, by ensuring your daily supplement programme contains 5,000IU (1,515mcg) of retinol. Vitamin A is also rich in fish and eggs.

See chapter 12 for more on supplements and also the Resources section for suppliers.

Immune power

Avoiding allergens is only half the story. The other half involves boosting your immune power to reduce allergic potential in the first place.

Lying on his deathbed, Louis Pasteur stated, 'The host is more important than the invader.' It's increasingly being recognised that we are more likely to succumb to bugs or allergies if we are run down, confirming the adage 'prevention is better than cure'. The best line of defence is to keep the immune system strong for when the next invader comes along. We are all exposed to germs that cause infectious diseases, but those of us with strong immune systems fight back more effectively and either avoid symptoms of the illness entirely or have a milder attack. This is especially key during pregnancy, when a virus or bug could harm your unborn baby.

Immune-boosting nutrients

Your immune strength is totally dependent on a sufficient supply of vitamins and minerals. Deficiencies of vitamins A, B1, B2, B5, B6, B12, folic acid, C and E suppress immunity, as do deficiencies of iron, zinc, magnesium and selenium. An optimal intake of these nutrients is vital in boosting immune strength.

Vitamin B1, B2 and B5 have mild immune-boosting effects compared with vitamin B6. The production of antibodies and other key immune cells, so critical in successfully fighting any infection, depends upon B6. Two other important B vitamins are B12 and folic acid. Both appear essential for proper immune function. B6, zinc and folic acid are all needed in the rapid production of new immune cells to engage an enemy.

Since no nutrients work in isolation, it's helpful to supplement a good high-strength multivitamin and mineral as well as eating an optimal diet – by following the Better Pregnancy Diet and Supplement Plan outlined in Part Two, you'll be doing this. The combination of nutrients in a multivitamin and mineral can have a strong effect on boosting immunity.

Extra help if you do get sick

If you do succumb to an infection while you're pregnant (or indeed at any time), the nutrients worth adding in larger amounts to help fight it off are the antioxidants and particularly vitamin C.

When your body is invaded by an infection, these invaders produce dangerous oxidising chemicals called 'free radicals' to weaken your immune system. Antioxidant nutrients such as vitamin A, C, E, zinc and selenium disarm these free radicals and turn the tables to weaken the invader. They also have a wide range of other immune-boosting functions. For example, vitamin A is especially important because it helps to maintain the integrity of the digestive tract, lungs and all cell membranes, preventing foreign agents from entering the body, or viruses from entering cells. Vitamin E is another important all-rounder. It improves immune cell function and is a powerful antioxidant. Selenium, iron, manganese, copper and zinc are all involved in antioxidation and have all been shown to positively affect immune power. So if your immune system needs a boost, supplement a daily antioxidant formula that contains these key ingredients (see the Resources section for a list of suppliers).

In addition, it's worth supplementing extra vitamin C. To date more than a dozen immune-boosting roles of vitamin C have been identified – it helps mature immune cells, improves their performance and is itself anti-viral and anti-bacterial, as well as being able to detoxify toxins produced by bacteria. In addition, it is a natural anti-histamine. However, the dosage of vitamin C is crucial. A review of studies looking at its protective effect against the common cold found that it was only consistently effective in doses of 1g or more (i.e. twenty times the RDA). So we suggest you take at least 1g of vitamin C daily, which you can increase to 2–3g every four hours if your immune system is under attack. The only word of caution is that large doses of vitamin C can cause loose bowels – but if this happens, just reduce the dose slightly until symptoms subside.

What about the flu jab?

If you're pregnant during the winter, your doctor may encourage you to have a flu vaccine. The reason is that while being pregnant puts you at no greater risk of catching influenza, you may suffer more complications such as pneumonia if you do. However, most flu jabs contain many toxic substances that could harm you and especially your vulnerable baby even more. For example, there may be thimerosal, a mercury-derived preservative, which can pass through the placenta and damage the developing brain and nervous system of your unborn baby (it can also harm older children and adults – see chapter 19 for more on vaccinations). The best way then to avoid flu is not to catch it in the first place, and you can increase your immunity by eating well and boosting your immune system with the key nutrients outlined in this chapter. Flu also spreads easily through coughing and sneezing. So wash your hands often and try to avoid crowds, especially groups of young children.

In summary, to banish allergies and boost immunity:

- **Play** detective and identify any possible allergens in the food you're eating, then eliminate any suspects and pulse test after fifteen days to check for a reaction.

- **Follow** any elimination diet with gut-healing nutrients such as Omega 3 fish oils, glutamine, vitamin A and zinc to repair any damage to your digestive tract. Also supplement digestive enzymes.

- **Boost** your immune system by following the nutrient-rich Better Pregnancy Diet and Supplement Plan, outlined in Part Two.

- **If** you feel your immune system needs a boost, or is under attack, supplement a daily antioxidant formula plus 1g of vitamin C, or more where required.

CHAPTER EIGHT

Essential Fats to Give Your Baby a Head Start

ID YOU KNOW that your intake of essential fats has a direct effect on your child's IQ? If you want to create a healthy, intelligent baby, eating the right kind of fats is absolutely vital. Like you, a baby's brain and nervous system are composed primarily of fats, and their hearts and blood vessels are also rich in fatty membranes. While it's important to ensure an adequate supply throughout life, there's no more important time than before and during pregnancy, when you need to provide the right building blocks for your baby to develop.

It's wise to start correcting any deficiency or imbalance in your essential fat status before you conceive, because not only are these fats needed for a healthy hormone balance (necessary to help you get pregnant in the first place), but it also takes time to correct any deficiency and build up optimum levels in your body. As soon as you become pregnant, your baby will need a good supply, especially in the crucial first three months of development when the brain and nervous and cardiovascular systems are forming.

The fats of life

Most people know that eating the wrong kinds of fat can lead to heart disease, cancer and obesity. But did you know that eating the right kind of fat not only reduces your risk of developing these diseases, it also protects against allergies, arthritis, eczema, depression, fatigue, infections and hormonal imbalances?

In a developing baby, essential fats (also called essential fatty acids or EFAs for short) are needed to construct the membranes of all cells and are particularly key to the development of brain and nerve tissue. In a pregnant mother, EFAs also help to maintain a healthy hormone balance, prevent pre-eclampsia (a condition where your blood pressure can become dangerously high – see page 135) and stop you having mood swings or post-natal depression. Then, once your baby is born, getting a good supply of EFAs from you via your milk can also protect them from developing food intolerances and allergies.

Yet despite all these crucial roles for EFAs in general health and pregnancy, many of us today are fat-phobic. And while we should be phobic about eating too much hard fat – found in dairy products, meat, processed foods and most margarines – restricting all fats means you are depriving yourself and your baby of essential health-giving nutrients and increasing your risk of poor health. In fact, unless you go out of your way to eat the right kind of fat-rich foods – such as seeds, nuts and fish – the chances are you're seriously deficient.

Fat figures

There are three kinds of fat: saturated, monounsaturated and polyunsaturated. Saturated and monounsaturated fat are not nutrients. You don't need them although they can be used by the body to make energy. Polyunsaturated fats or oils are essential.

Almost all foods that contain fat are made up of a balance of all three. A piece of meat, for example, will have mainly saturated and monounsaturated fat with a little polyunsaturated fat. Olive oil has mainly monounsaturated fat. Sunflower seed oil has mainly polyun-saturated fat.

Most authorities now agree that, of our total fat intake, no more than one-third should be saturated (hard) fat and at least one-third

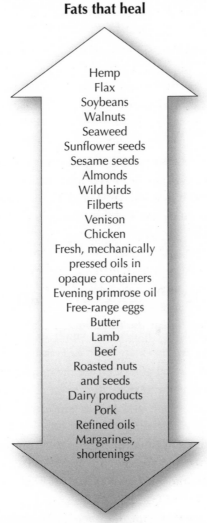

Fats that heal

Hemp
Flax
Soybeans
Walnuts
Seaweed
Sunflower seeds
Sesame seeds
Almonds
Wild birds
Filberts
Venison
Chicken
Fresh, mechanically
pressed oils in
opaque containers
Evening primrose oil
Free-range eggs
Butter
Lamb
Beef
Roasted nuts
and seeds
Dairy products
Pork
Refined oils
Margarines,
shortenings

Fats that kill

Fats that heal, fats that kill

should be polyunsaturated oils providing two kinds of essential fats: the linoleic acid family, known as Omega 6; and the alpha-linolenic acid family, known as Omega 3 (more on these later). Monounsaturated fats make up the other third.

The ideal balance between Omega 3 and 6 is about twice as much 6 to 3. So an ideal 'fat profile', based on fat forming no more than 20 per cent of our total calorie intake, might consist of:

- 4 per cent Omega 6

- 3 per cent Omega 3

- 7 per cent monounsaturated fat

- 6 per cent saturated fat.

Most people are deficient in Omega 3 and good quality Omega 6 fats. In addition, a high intake of saturated fats and damaged polyunsaturated fats, known as 'trans' fats (found in processed or fried foods), stops the body making good use of the little essential fats the average person eats in a day.

The 'Omega 6' fat family

The grandmother of the Omega-6 fat family is linoleic acid. Linoleic acid is converted by the body into gamma-linolenic acid (GLA). Evening primrose oil and borage oil are the richest known sources of GLA and, by supplementing these direct you need take in less overall fat to get an optimal intake of Omega 6. The ideal intake during pregnancy and while breast feeding is around 200mg of GLA a day, which is equivalent to about 2,500mg of evening primrose oil, or 1,000mg of high-potency borage oil – one or two capsules a day.

GLA then gets converted into DGLA (di-homo gamma linolenic acid) and from there into 'prostaglandins', which are extremely active, hormone-like substances in the body. The particular kind of prostaglandins made from these Omega 6 oils is called 'Series 1 prostaglandins'. These keep the blood thin, relax blood vessels, lower blood pressure, help to maintain water balance in the body, decrease inflammation and pain, improve nerve and immune function and help insulin to work, which is good for blood glucose balance – all essential during pregnancy. And this is the short-list. As every year passes more and more health-promoting functions are being found. Prostaglandins themselves cannot be supplemented as they are very short-lived. Instead we rely on a good intake of Omega 6 fats from which the body can make the prostaglandins we need.

A deficiency of Omega 6 fats in pregnancy can seriously impact on your baby's health – after birth he or she may fail to thrive, suffer with diarrhoea, skin problems, poor hair growth and poor utilisation of food for energy.

Omega 6 Deficiency Signs

Yes No

☐ ☐ Do you have high blood pressure?

☐ ☐ Do you suffer from PMS or breast pain?

☐ ☐ Do you suffer from eczema or dry skin?

☐ ☐ Do you suffer from dry eyes?

☐ ☐ Do you have an inflammatory health problem, like arthritis?

☐ ☐ Do you have difficulty losing weight?

☐ ☐ Do you have a blood glucose problem or diabetes?

☐ ☐ Do you have multiple sclerosis?

☐ ☐ Do you drink alcohol every day?

☐ ☐ Do you have any mental health problems?

☐ ☐ Do you suffer from excessive thirst?

How do you score? Five or more 'yes' answers indicates that you may be deficient in Omega 6 fats. Check your diet carefully for the seeds and oils listed on page 80.

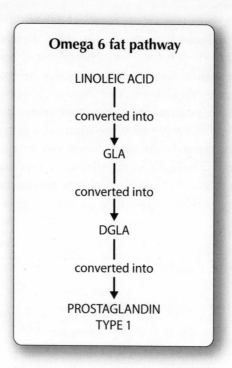

Omege 6 fat pathway

This family of fats comes exclusively from seeds and their oils. The best seed oils are hemp, pumpkin, sunflower, safflower, sesame, corn, walnut, and soya bean and wheatgerm oil. About half of the fats in these oils comes from the Omega 6 family, mainly as linoleic acid. An optimal intake would be about one to two tablespoons or capsules of an Omega 6 oil a day, plus two to three tablespoons of ground seeds (or, as outlined earlier, one or two capsules of evening primrose or borage oil).

The 'Omega 3' fat family

The modern diet is likely to be even more deficient in Omega 3 fats than Omega 6 fats simply because the grandmother of the Omega 3 family, alpha-linolenic acid, and her metabolically active grand-children, EPA (eicosapentaenoic acid) and DHA (docosahexaenoic acid), are more prone to damage in cooking and food processing. It is from EPA and DHA that Series 3 prostaglandins are made.

Series 3 prostaglandins are essential for proper brain function, affecting vision, learning ability, coordination and mood. They also reduce the stickiness of blood, as well as controlling blood cholesterol and fat levels, improve immune function and metabolism, reducing inflammation and maintain water balance. So they are not only vital for your health before, during and after pregnancy, but also for the health of your future baby.

Omega 3 fats for a brainy baby

As Omega 3 fats are so key in brain development, a deficiency during pregnancy can lead to permanent learning disabilities.[91] Conversely, a good supply during pregnancy can increase a baby's brainpower. The Omega 3 fat DHA is particularly rich in cod liver oil. In a study of 300 women given either a cod liver oil or corn oil (effectively a placebo) supplement during pregnancy and for three months following birth, the intelligence of their children was tested once they reached the age of four. Children born to mothers in the cod liver oil group scored higher in the tests, which gauged problem solving and information processing abilities.[92] DHA is important for mental performance and plays a key role in the growth of your developing baby's brain and nervous system. It's also produced in breast milk, so after your baby is born, as long as you eat a good supply yourself, he or she will continue to have a good source.

Fish oil prevents premature birth

Fish oils can also prevent premature birth and low birth-weight. A study of nearly 9,000 pregnant women in Denmark found that those who ate no fish were around three times more likely to have a premature delivery than those who did. Overall, women who ate some fish were less likely than those who did not to deliver prematurely, and their babies tended to weigh more. For example, the rate of premature birth among women who ate no fish was about 7 per cent, compared with roughly 2 per cent for women who had fish at least once a week.[93]

Omega 3 fats reduce depression

A good supply of Omega 3 fats can prevent depression during and after pregnancy. In a study of 11,721 British women, researchers found that those who consumed greater amounts of seafood during the third trimester of their pregnancy were less likely to show signs of major depression before and for up to eight months after the birth. Women with the highest intakes of Omega 3, who consumed fish two or three times a week, were half as likely to suffer from depression as women with the lowest intakes.[94]

Sadly, oily fish – a rich source of Omega 3 fats – is often polluted, so while sardines, organic or wild Pacific salmon and mackerel or herring from unpolluted seas are the best options, you can also ensure you get a good supply of these essential fats by taking a 'pure' fish oil supplement (see page 84 for more details).

Omega 3 deficiency signs

Yes No

☐ ☐ Do you have dry skin?

☐ ☐ Do you have any inflammatory health problems, such as asthma, dermatitis or eczema?

☐ ☐ Do you suffer from water retention?

☐ ☐ Do you get tingling in the arms or legs?

☐ ☐ Do you have high blood pressure or high triglycerides?

☐ ☐ Are you prone to infections?

☐ ☐ Are you finding it hard to lose weight?

☐ ☐   Have your memory and learning ability declined?

☐ ☐   Do you suffer from a lack of coordination or impaired vision?

How do you score? Five or more 'yes' answers indicates that you may be deficient in omega 3 fats. Check your diet carefully for the foods listed below.

The best seed oils for Omega 3 fats are flax (also known as linseed), hemp and pumpkin. Eating carnivorous fish or their oils provides a more direct source of the Omega 3 fats EPA and DHA (see the 'Omega 3 pathway', above). This is why fish eaters like the Japanese have three times the Omega 3 fats in their body fat than the average American. Vegans, who eat more seeds and nuts, have twice the Omega 3 fat level than the average American.

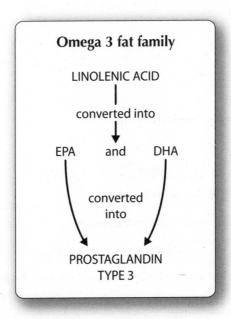

Omega 3 pathway

Essential Omegas

The easiest way to get a good daily balance of essential fats before, during and after pregnancy (and while breast feeding) is to (a) have one heaped tablespoon of ground mixed seeds or cold-pressed seed oils, and (b) take a supplement that provides 400mg of EPA, 200mg of DHA and 200mg of GLA (see the Resources section for suppliers). This way, you ensure you cover all the bases to ensure a good mix of all the essential fats you and your developing baby need.

To make an Omega 3/6-rich seed mix, put one measure each of sesame, sunflower and pumpkin seeds and two measures of flax seeds in a sealed jar and keep it in the fridge, away from light, heat and oxygen. Then grind some of the mixture fresh each day, using a food or coffee grinder, and add a heaped tablespoon to your breakfast each morning. Alternatively, dress a salad, baked potato or steamed vegetables with a tablespoon of cold-pressed seed oil.

Of these seeds, the most unsaturated is flax and hence it is the most prone to damage. For this reason it's important to buy fresh seeds that have been properly stored, minimising heat, light and oxygen exposure. A small number of companies offer seed oils that are processed in such a way as to protect the oils from oxidation, thus preserving their essential fat status. We recommend you only buy oils that are extracted from organic seeds, cold-pressed to minimise heat, and stored in a light-proof container.

Phospholipids: the smart fats

Phospholipids are a type of 'intelligent' polyunsaturated fat found in our brains. They are the insulation experts, helping signals in the brain to run smoothly because they make up the insulating layer, or myelin, around all nerves. There are several different types of phospholipids, but in pregnancy, phosphidtyl choline has been identified as particularly important for your baby's brain development.

Recent research has shown that supplementing phosphidtyl choline during pregnancy can create a 'superbrain' in the baby. This research, carried out at Duke University Medical Center in the US, fed pregnant rats choline halfway through their pregnancy. Once they were born, the infant rats had vastly superior brains, improved learning ability and better memory recall, all of which continued into old age. The research showed that giving phosphidtyl choline helps restructure the brain for improved performance. Supplementing choline in adults has also shown to boost memory.[95]

The richest source of phospholipids in the average diet is egg yolks. But not all eggs are created equal. While battery farmed eggs are often rich in bad fats and cholesterol, a brand of egg called Columbus is rich in good fats and phospholipids because the hens are fed a diet of flax seeds. You can buy Columbus eggs from most good UK supermarkets – aim to eat five to seven a week during pregnancy to boost levels of phosphidtyl choline. Lecithin is also a rich source of phosphidtyl choline, and you can buy this in granules from your health food shop to sprinkle daily on cereal or in soups. How much you need will depend on the phospholipid content – with most brands, about a tablespoon should do it, or if you buy 'Hi-PC' lecithin, you'll only need a teaspoon. See Resources section for more details.

The dangers of trans-fats

Refining and processing vegetable oils can change the nature of the polyunsaturated oil. An example of this is the making of margarine. To turn the vegetable oil into a hard fat the oil is 'hydrogenated'. Although the fat is still technically polyunsaturated the body cannot make use of it. Even worse than that, it blocks the body's ability to use healthy polyunsaturated oils and raises cholesterol levels. This is called a 'trans' fat because it has been changed. It's like a key that fits the body's chemical locks but won't open the door. Most margarines contain these 'hydrogenated polyunsaturated oils' and are best avoided. So too are foods containing hydrogenated fats such as biscuits, cakes and ready meals, so check the label carefully.

Research has found that as well as blocking the functions of essential fats, too many trans-fats can also disrupt pregnancy hormones, reduce a baby's birth-weight and lower the quality of breast milk, as well as decreasing testosterone and increasing abnormal sperm in men.[96,97] So to minimise your risks, try to steer clear of hydrogenated margarines (look for makes free of hydrogenated fats, or use butter in moderation) and processed foods.

Frying is another way to damage otherwise healthy oils. The high temperature makes the oil oxidise and so, instead of being good for you, oxidised or rancid oils generate harmful 'free radicals' in the body. Frying is therefore best avoided as is any form of burning or browning fat. However, if you do fry use a tiny amount of olive oil or butter, since these are less prone to oxidation than top-quality, cold-pressed vegetable oils. These cold-pressed oils should be kept sealed in the fridge, away from heat, light and oxygen, and used for 'cold' purposes only such as salad dressings or spreads, or instead of butter on your baked potato or peas.

The general guidelines for getting the right kind and amount of fat in your diet are:

- **Eat** two tablespoons of freshly ground mixed seeds (sesame, sunflower, pumpkin and flax) or just one tablespoon of ground seeds plus one tablespoon of cold-pressed seed oil per day.

- **Eat** oily fish such as sardines, organic salmon and mackerel or herring from unpolluted seas at least once, and preferably three times a week, or take a daily fish oil supplement (see page 84).

- **Avoid** fried food, burnt or browned fat, saturated and 'hydrogenated' fat.

- **If** you do fry use olive oil or butter, and do so as little as possible.

- **To** boost levels of phospholipids, have five to seven free-range eggs, such as Columbus, a week, or put a tablespoon of lecithin granules on your cereal each day.

PART TWO

THE PERFECT PREGNANCY PLAN

Congratulations! Now you're expecting a baby. This section will show you:

- The best sources of protein, fats and carbohydrate to nourish optimally both you and your growing baby.

- Why vitamins and minerals are vital for your baby's development and how they keep you vibrant and healthy.

- Meal plans with ideas for delicious food to enjoy.

- Why taking supplements is essential.

- How to prevent common pregnancy problems, from anaemia to weight gain.

- The secrets of keeping energised and feeling on top form.

- How to exercise safely to be fighting fit for the big day.

CHAPTER NINE

~

Optimum Nutrition for a Healthy Pregnancy

B ABIES DEMAND THE best and no time is more important for optimum nutrition than while you're pregnant. Even if your diet was adequate before you conceived, you can't assume it will continue to meet your (and your baby's) needs for the next nine months. In fact, most people who think they eat a 'well-balanced diet' fail to meet even the basic RDA level of nutrients. At any time of bodily stress – and this includes puberty, menopause, menstruation, but most of all pregnancy – nutritional needs are greatest. All your resources will be called upon and if you don't have enough nutrients in the bank, you'll go overdrawn.

What does this mean? Well, medical evidence suggests that babies who have to adapt to a limited supply of nutrients while developing in the womb permanently change their underlying physiology and metabolism. Even if they are born seemingly 'healthy', these adaptations are the origins of most degenerative diseases in later life.[1] And mothers who are deficient are more likely to develop health problems during and after pregnancy – for example stretch marks and post-natal depression are both signs of zinc deficiency. But you can prevent all this by having a better pregnancy diet, which boosts your intake of the many essential nutrients you and your growing baby need. Before we look at what that means in terms of what you actually eat, let's first consider what the building blocks of a healthy diet are, kicking off with the 'macro' nutrients – protein, fat and carbohydrate.

Protein: the body's building blocks

The word protein is derived from 'protos', meaning 'first' since protein is the basic material of all living cells. The human body is, for example, approximately 65 per cent water and 25 per cent protein. As well as being vital for growth and the repair of body tissue, protein is used to make hormones, enzymes, antibodies, and neurotransmitters, and helps transport substances around the body.

While protein forms the building blocks of the body, amino acids are the building blocks of protein. Some twenty-two different types of amino acids are pieced together in different combinations to make various kinds of protein, in much the same way as letters make words, which combine to make sentences and paragraphs. Of these twenty-two, sixteen can be made by your body, but the remaining eight must come from your diet. These eight are therefore termed 'essential' and their balance in the protein of any given food determines its quality, or usability.

During pregnancy, your need for protein increases as you are not just replenishing your own body, but also providing the raw materials from which your baby is made. As a result, the UK recommended intake for protein goes up by 13 per cent – from 45g a day (or 15 per cent of total calories) to around 51g.[2] However, this allows for a big safety margin and doesn't mean you must eat lots of steaks, eggs or cheese to get what you need. The belief that you can only get good-quality protein from animal products is a myth. The best quality protein foods in terms of amino acid balance include quinoa (a South American grain, pronounced 'keen-wah'), soya, fish, beans and lentils, as well as meat, eggs and dairy products. What's more, animal protein sources tend to contain a lot of undesirable saturated fat, whereas vegetable protein sources often contain additional beneficial complex carbohydrates (see later) and are less acid-forming than meat.

Acid is a by-product of protein metabolism and too much is not good because minerals such as calcium and magnesium – both essential, especially during pregnancy – are then used to buffer the acidity, and therefore cannot be used to keep bones strong or muscles healthy. This is why frequent meat eaters have a higher risk of osteoporosis.[3]

So you don't need to rely on animal sources to meet your protein needs. As well as fish, grains, pulses, soya, nuts and seeds, many vegetables – especially 'seed' foods such as runner beans, peas, corn or broccoli – contain good levels of protein and also help to neutralise excess acidity.

Packed with protein: the top 24

Food	Percentage of calories as protein	How much for 20g protein	Protein quality (NPU)
Grains/pulses			
Quinoa	16	100g/3½ oz/1 cup dry weight	Excellent
Tofu	40	275g/10 oz/1 packet	Reasonable
Corn	4	500g/1 lb 2 oz/3 cups cooked weight	Reasonable
Brown rice	5	400g/14 oz/3 cups cooked weight	Excellent
Chickpeas	22	115g/4 oz/⅔ cup cooked weight	Reasonable
Lentils	28	85g/3 oz/1 cup cooked weight	Reasonable
Fish/meat			
Tuna, canned	61	85g/3 oz/1 small can	Excellent
Cod	60	35g/1½ oz/1 very small piece	Excellent
Salmon	50	100g/3½ oz/ 1 very small piece	Excellent
Sardines	49	100g/3½ oz/ 1 grilled	Excellent
Chicken	63	75g/2½ oz/1 small roasted breast	Excellent
Nuts/seeds			
Sunflower seeds	15	185g/6½ oz/1 cup	Reasonable

Food	Percentage of calories as protein	How much for 20g protein	Protein quality (NPU)
Pumpkin seeds	21	75g/2½ oz/½ cup	Reasonable
Cashew nuts	12	115g/4 oz/1 cup	Reasonable
Almonds	13	115g/4 oz/1 cup	Reasonable
Eggs/dairy			
Eggs	34	115g/4 oz/2 medium	Excellent
Yoghurt, natural	22	450g/1 lb/3 small pots	Excellent
Cottage cheese	49	125g/4½ oz/1 small pot	Excellent
Vegetables			
Peas, frozen	26	250g/9 oz/2 cups	Reasonable
Other beans	20	200g/7 oz/2 cups	Reasonable
Broccoli	50	40g/1½ oz/½ cup	Reasonable
Spinach	49	40g/1½ oz/⅔ cup	Reasonable
Combinations			
Lentils and rice	18	125g/4½ oz/small cup dry weight	Excellent
Beans and rice	15	125g/4½ oz/small cup dry weight	Excellent

How big is a serving?

When you need to know how much one portion or serving size is, use this as a general guide:

Grains (cooked pasta, rice, oats, cereal) – the size of a tennis ball
Bread – one slice or half a roll or bagel
Cheese – one-and-a-half thumbs' worth
Fish/meat – the size of a deck of playing cards or a small woman's palm
Butter – one teaspoon or the size of the tip of your thumb
Fruit and vegetables
Standard fruit (apple, pear, orange) – one fruit
Small fruit (plums, apricots, satsumas) – two fruits
Very large fruit (melon, pineapple) – one large slice

Berries (raspberries, strawberries, grapes) – one teacup full

Fresh fruit salad, tinned or stewed fruit – three heaped tablespoons

Dried fruit (currants, sultanas, figs) – one heaped tablespoonful

Fruit juice (preferably fresh juice) – one small glass

Vegetables (raw, cooked or frozen) – two heaped tablespoons

Salad – a dessert bowl or two cupped hands full

Good and bad fats

As explained in chapter 8, there are two main kinds of fats: saturated (hard) fat and unsaturated fat. It is neither essential to eat saturated fat, nor ideal to eat too much. The main sources are meat and dairy products. There are also two kinds of unsaturated fats: monounsaturated fats, rich in olive oil; and polyunsaturated fats, found in nuts, seeds and their oils and fish, which are essential for both you and your baby.

The optimal diet – whether you are pregnant or not – provides a balance of these two essential polyunsaturated fats, also known as Omega 3 and Omega 6 oils. Pumpkin and flax seeds are rich in linolenic acid (Omega 3), while sesame and sunflower seeds are rich in linoleic acid (Omega 6). Linolenic acid is converted in the body into DHA and EPA, which are also found in mackerel, herring, salmon and sardines.

These essential fats are easily destroyed by heating or exposure to oxygen, so having a fresh daily source is important. See Chapter 8 for how easy it is to incorporate these into your daily diet. Processed foods often contain hardened or 'hydrogenated' polyunsaturated fats and these are worse for you than saturated fat and are best avoided (see page 85 for more on this).

Carbohydrates: the sweet truth

The human body is designed to run on carbohydrates. While we can use protein and fat for energy, the easiest and most 'smoke-free' fuel is carbohydrate. Plants make carbohydrate by trapping the sun's energy in a complex of carbon, hydrogen and oxygen. We eat the carbohydrate and, in the presence of oxygen from the air we breathe, break it down and release the stored solar energy, which then provides energy for our body and mind.

When you eat 'complex' carbohydrates like wholegrains, vegetables, beans or lentils, or simpler carbohydrates such as fruit, the body does exactly what it's designed to do. It digests these foods and gradually releases their potential energy. What's more, all the nutrients the body needs for digestion and metabolism are present in those whole foods that can literally be plucked out of a tree or pulled from the ground. These foods also contain a less digestible type of carbohydrate, classified as fibre, which helps keep the digestive system running smoothly.

Humankind has, however, learnt to cheat nature by isolating the sweetness in food and discarding the rest. All forms of concentrated sugar, such as white sugar, brown sugar, malt, glucose, honey and syrup, are 'fast releasing', causing a rapid increase in blood sugar levels. The way the body responds to a sudden onslaught of sugar in the blood is to take it out into the cells. If they don't need more fuel the sugar is put into storage, first as 'glycogen' in muscles and the liver, then as fat (yes, that means too much sugar makes you fat!). Most concentrated forms of sugar are also devoid of vitamins and minerals, unlike the natural sources, such as fruit. White sugar has around 90 per cent of its vitamins and minerals removed. Without vitamins and minerals, your metabolism becomes inefficient, contributing to poor energy and poor weight control.

Refined carbohydrates such as white bread, white rice or refined cereals have a similar effect to refined sugar. The process of refining or even cooking starts to break down complex carbohydrates into simple carbohydrates, in effect pre-digesting them. When you eat them you get a rapid increase in blood sugar level and a corresponding surge in energy. The surge, however, is followed by a drop as the body scrambles to balance your blood sugar level.

When you're pregnant, your carbohydrate intake has to meet not just your energy needs, but also those of your baby. As your baby is growing around the clock, their need is constant. So fluctuations in blood sugar levels are likely to cause a more pronounced reaction. Feeling dizzy, irritable, forgetful, jittery, tired or thirsty are all signs of low blood sugar. And while it's easy to respond by reaching for some chocolate, biscuits or a cup of coffee, this just creates a vicious cycle of sugar surges followed by sugar lows, which not only makes you feel like you're on an energy roller-coaster, but can lead to gestational diabetes (see page 132). A very high intake of refined sugar can also interfere with normal glucose metabolism and this can lead to birth defects.[4]

The answer is to eat small, frequent meals containing either some protein or complex carbohydrate. Snack on sunflower seeds, nuts, oatcakes and slow-releasing fruit, such as apples, cherries or oranges, rather than biscuits, sweets and cakes. Dilute fruit juices with water as these are fairly high in natural sugars and watch out for satisfying your sweet tooth by eating loads of dried fruit or honey under the guise that you've stopped eating sugar. See chapter 14 for more tips on balancing your blood sugar.

Fibre: keeping things moving

Fibre is a key part of our diets, not because it contributes any specific nutrients itself, but because it slows down their absorption (therefore helping to balance blood sugar) and makes the contents of our digestive tracts bulkier and easier to pass through. It also helps to prevent constipation and putrefaction of foods, which can be underlying causes of many digestive complaints.

This is especially important during pregnancy as constipation and wind are common problems. As your baby grows, he or she will press on your abdomen, making it harder for you to eat a lot and providing less room for digested waste to be passed out for elimination. If your diet is high in sticky, mucousy foods such as meat and milk and low in fibre-rich foods such as vegetables and wholegrains, your stools become more and more compact and harder to pass. In fact the word constipation comes from the Latin word *constipare*, meaning to pack together.

High fibre doesn't mean just adding bran to a fibre-poor diet. It is far better to get your fibre from the foods you eat. All vegetables, grains, nuts, lentils and beans contain significant amounts of fibre. Oats, linseeds and brown rice are particularly fibre-rich and gentler than wheat bran, which can be abrasive to the digestive tract. Also choose wholegrains and wholemeal bread instead of white rice, pasta, bread, etc. And drink lots of water, which is needed for fibre to absorb to bulk up and soften waste matter.

To get the best sources of protein, fat, carbohydrate and fibre during pregnancy, follow these simple guidelines:

- **Eat** 2 servings of beans, lentils, quinoa, tofu (soya), 'seed' vegetables or other vegetable protein, and 1 small serving of meat, fish, cheese or a free-range egg a day.

- **Avoid** excess protein from animal sources.

- **Eat** 2 tablespoons of ground seeds a day or 1 plus 1 tablespoon of cold-pressed seed oil (i.e. flax seed or hemp oil).

- **Avoid** fried food, burnt or browned fat, saturated and 'hydrogenated' fat.

- **Eat** 3 or more servings of dark green, leafy and root vegetables such as watercress, carrots, sweet potatoes, broccoli, Brussels sprouts, spinach, green beans or peppers, raw or lightly cooked.

- **Eat** 3 or more servings of fresh fruit such as apples, pears, bananas, berries, melon or citrus fruit.

- **Eat** 4 or more servings of wholegrains such as rice, millet, rye, oats, wholewheat, corn, quinoa as cereal, breads, pasta or pulses.

- **Avoid** any form of sugar, foods with added sugar, white or refined foods.

CHAPTER TEN

The A–Z of Essential Nutrients

VITAMINS AND MINERALS are needed in much smaller amounts than fat, protein or carbohydrate, hence they are known as 'micronutrients'. However, they are no less important, especially during pregnancy. This is because vitamins and minerals are the keys that make enzymes kick into action in the body. Enzymes are what do the work in your body, turning one substance into another. For example, to digest protein into amino acids, and then build proteins for your baby, you need enzymes. They are the catalysts that make all body processes happen. These vital nutrients are therefore needed to balance hormones, produce energy, boost the immune system, build bones and teeth, make healthy skin and protect the arteries. They are vital for the brain, nervous system and more... They are involved in just about every function of the body. If you're deficient, your body simply won't work as efficiently as it could. But if your baby doesn't get enough, key organs won't develop properly, resulting in lifelong disability. So let's consider what specific vitamins and minerals do, what quantity you need and where you can get a good source from diet and supplements.

The recommended daily allowance (RDA)

For nearly all nutrients – from protein to vitamins and minerals – governments set a 'recommended daily allowance' (RDA) or 'reference nutrient intake' (RNI) as a guideline to what the general population should be getting. These levels are designed to prevent you developing nutritional deficiency diseases such as scurvy or rickets. However, there is a big difference between an absence of disease and an abundance of health. For example, the average person gets three-and-a-half colds a year. Yet, in a study of 1,038 doctors and their wives, those with an intake of 410mg of vitamin C a day had the least signs of illness and lowest incidence of colds. This intake is roughly ten times the RDA for vitamin C. There is also a large discrepancy between the RDA levels set by different governments. In the US, for example, the RDA of minerals for pregnant women is between 14 and 100 per cent higher than the British RNI equivalent.[5] And while pregnancy obviously merits an increased intake, there are no additional allowances suggested if you live in a polluted city, are under stress, exercise a lot or have an infection – all of which increase your nutrient requirement further, some by as much as double again. So while the RDA or RNI is a basic guideline, it's far below the level we suggest you aim for if you want to be in optimum health, especially while you're pregnant.

Vital vitamins

Vitamins fall into two categories – water soluble or fat soluble. The water-soluble ones are the B vitamins (of which there are eight main types), vitamin C and vitamin K – levels of these need replenishing daily. Vitamins A, D and E are fat soluble and are stored in your body fat, so although you need to maintain a good intake, it's not so essential to ensure this is as regular as water-soluble nutrients.

For most nutrients, you will see that as well as eating plenty of the right food sources, you also need to supplement to reach the levels you need, and this is explored in more detail in chapter 12. Where we refer to RDAs, we are quoting American levels rather than European RDAs or their UK-equivalent RNIs as these are more comprehensive (although still often far below what we have found to be optimal – see the 'Recommended daily allowance' box above for more on this).

Vitamin A: essential for growth

Vitamin A is a fat-soluble vitamin found in both animal foods (where it's called retinol) and some vegetables (betacarotene). Retinol is the 'active' form and is especially rich in liver,* since this is where it is stored in the body (hence cod liver oil is a popular source). It is commonly measured in international units (or 'IU') and more recently in micrograms ('mcg').

What it does

Vitamin A is vital for proper growth in your baby and plays an important part in his or her visual and hearing development, as well as proper heart and immune functions. In you, vitamin A is important for healthy skin, a strong immune system (including protection against cancer) and is essential for night vision.

How much do I need?

There is some controversy over vitamin A during pregnancy. But there's no doubt that it's essential – you just don't want too much. The optimum level is around 2,275mcg (7,500IU). Anything over 3,000mcg (10,000IU) is not recommended for women of childbearing age, in case they conceive, unless given under the supervision of a nutritional therapist or knowledgeable doctor. See chapter 5 for further details.

Best food sources: beef liver,* veal liver,* carrots, watercress, cabbage, squash, sweet potato, melon, pumpkin, mangoes, tomato, broccoli, apricots, papayas, tangerines and asparagus.

* See page 120 re. caution in eating liver during pregnancy

Best supplement: retinol (animal source) and natural betacarotene or retinyl palmitate (vegetable source). Zinc is needed to convert betacarotene into the active form of vitamin A, retinol. Best taken with food as part of a multivitamin and mineral supplement or antioxidant formula.

B vitamins: the energy nutrients

The family of B vitamins includes vitamins B1, B2, B3, B5, B6, B12 plus biotin and perhaps the best-known nutrient in pregnancy, folic acid. While each one has specific functions, they mostly work together so you need a good balance of all eight.

What they do

The B vitamins create new blood cells for your growing baby and are key for brain development and cell division, which is obviously important in the first few months of pregnancy. Vitamin B6 is especially key in your baby's developing nervous system, while together with B12 and folic acid, it keeps homocysteine low (see chapter 6) and prevents birth defects such as cleft palate and spina bifida (see chapter 5). This trio, along with zinc, keep homocysteine levels low in you too and work with the rest of the B vitamin family to produce energy. They also maintain healthy skin, hair and a healthy hormone balance (a deficiency of B6, for example, is common in PMS sufferers).

How much do I need?

Even eating an optimal diet will rarely provide the right balance of every B vitamin in optimal quantities. But the amounts included in a good multivitamin and mineral supplement should top you up to the right level. As a rough guide, aim to supplement around:

- 20–25mg of B1, B2, B3 and B5

- 50mg of B6, B12 and biotin

- 600mcg of folic acid.

Best food sources: mushrooms, watercress, cabbage, cauliflower, broccoli, alfalfa sprouts, squash, tomatoes (B1, B2, B3, B5, B6, biotin); chicken and salmon (B3); sardines, lamb, eggs and cottage cheese (B12); bananas (B6); nuts and seeds (folic acid).

Best supplement: B complex or within a multivitamin and mineral, as B6 works best with zinc and all work with the minerals magnesium and manganese.

Vitamin C: keeping skin firm

Vitamin C has so many roles in pregnancy it's hard to know where to start. Our need is also constant, so it's best to eat vitamin-C-rich foods throughout the day and take supplements in two separate doses.

What it does

Vitamin C is essential for the formation of collagen, which, among other things, helps to keep the protective membrane surrounding your baby strong. Collagen also keeps your bones, skin and joints firm, and helps to keep skin supple, which is vital for preventing stretch marks. Vitamin C is an important antioxidant, detoxifying pollutants and protecting against cancer and heart disease. It's also key for a healthy immune system.

How much do I need?

Your need increases during pregnancy and we believe a daily intake of at least 1,500–2,000mg is optimal, rather than the paltry RDA of just 70mg. To compensate for any dietary shortfall, we recommend you supplement at least 1,000mg, and more if you are stressed or live in a polluted environment.

Best food sources: peppers, watercress, cabbage, broccoli, cauliflower, strawberries, lemons, kiwi fruit, peas, melons, oranges, grapefruit, limes, tomatoes.

Best supplement: vitamin C can be mildly acidic in the digestive tract and in large doses (5,000mg plus). The ascorbate form (e.g. calcium ascorbate, magnesium ascorbate) or Ester C are mildly alkaline and more easily tolerated. Vitamin C works with bioflavanoids and good supplements include these. As we recommend you take more vitamin C than a multivitamin will provide, you will need to take an additional supplement.

Vitamin D: the bone builder

Unlike any other vitamin, vitamin D can be made in the skin in the presence of sunlight. Hence it is very difficult to become completely deficient. Vitamin D deficiency is not common in Britain, except in pregnant vegetarian Asian women, who, for reasons of skin colour, filter out the sun's ultraviolet rays and produce less vitamin D.

What it does

During pregnancy, your need for vitamin D increases as it is key for your baby's growth and bone development as well as the formation of tooth enamel (your baby's first teeth are already partly formed before he or she is born), so it is essential to get some from your diet and supplements as well. In you, vitamin D helps maintain strong and healthy bones by retaining calcium.

How much do I need?

The UK government recommends pregnant women supplement 10mcg a day. We recommend you get 120mcg (especially if you are pregnant in the winter), with 60mcg from a supplement.

Best food sources: herring, mackerel, salmon, cottage cheese, eggs.

Best supplement: cholecalciferol (animal origin) and ergocalciferol (yeast origin). Best taken as a multivitamin, as vitamins A, C and E protect D.

Vitamin K: vital for blood clotting

What it does

Vitamin K is called the clotting factor because it is involved in the manufacture of a protein called prothrombin, which makes your blood clot. Normally it's manufactured by bacteria in the gut. However, a baby's gut is sterile after birth and must rely on the mother's supply. Breast milk contains a factor that inhibits vitamin K so breast-feeding mothers need to take special care to eat enough cauliflower and cabbage, which are high in vitamin K. Although very rare, unexplained bleeding in young infants can be due to vitamin K deficiency. This is why after you give birth, a vitamin K injection is likely be offered to your baby. But as long as you're getting a good dietary supply and intend on breast feeding, there is no need for this (see page 157).

How much do I need?

Sufficient amounts should be made by beneficial bacteria in the gut, but also ensure a good intake of dietary sources while pregnant.

Best food sources: cauliflower, Brussels sprouts, lettuce, cabbage, beans, broccoli, peas, watercress, asparagus, potatoes.

Best supplement: not necessary to supplement if you have healthy intestinal bacteria (see pages 127–8, 'Family history of allergies?', for more on this).

Vitamin E: protecting cells

What it does

Like vitamin C, E helps get oxygen to the cells and protects the vital RNA and DNA (the genetic material in each body cell) from damage which could result in congenital defects for your baby. It also speeds up wound healing and helps to keep skin supple. It is particularly useful if applied externally for those who give birth by Caesarean section – we have seen scars completely disappear with topical application of vitamin E.

How much do I need?

The optimum level in pregnancy is 270mg (400IU) per day. A good diet will provide about 13.4mg (20IU), so top this up with a supplement providing 255mg (380IU).

Best food sources: sunflower seeds, peanuts, sesame seeds and other 'seed' foods, such as beans, peas, wheatgerm, and sardines, salmon and sweet potatoes.

Best supplement: d-alpha tocopherol (not synthetic dl-alpha tocopherol) as part of a multi or antioxidant supplement.

Magic minerals

Just as important as vitamins, and perhaps even more frequently deficient, are minerals. These are mainly used to regulate and balance our body chemistry, with the exception of calcium, phosphorus and magnesium, which are the major constituents of bone. These three, plus sodium and potassium – which control the water balance in the body – are called 'macro minerals' because we need relatively large amounts each day (300mg to 3,000mg). The remaining elements are called 'trace minerals' because we need only traces (30mcg to 30mg). For instance, you need around 1,200mg of calcium a day when you are pregnant, but only 40mcg of chromium (0.04mg). Yet chromium is no less important.

Calcium: vital for bones and teeth

What it does

Calcium is a vital component of your baby's bones and teeth and promotes a healthy heart and nervous system. In you, too, it's necessary for healthy bones, teeth and skin, as well as relieving aching muscles.

How much do I need?

When you're pregnant, your body absorbs more calcium from your diet than normal. But you still need to ensure you're getting about 1,200mg per day, which is more than double the average intake and almost impossible to get without supplementing.

Best food sources: Swiss cheese, cheddar cheese, almonds, parsley, corn tortillas, globe artichoke, dried prunes, pumpkin seeds, cooked dried beans, cabbage. Green leafy vegetables contain a balanced calcium to magnesium ratio and meat and poultry supply phosphorus necessary for calcium to function.

Best supplement: calcium is reasonably well absorbed in any form, but the best supplements contain calcium amino acid chelate or citrate (both approximately twice as well absorbed as calcium carbonate). A multi should supply most of what you need; check your chosen brand against the table in chapter 12 and, if necessary, take an additional supplement. As calcium works in partnership with magnesium, it's vital to take one that's balanced two parts calcium to one part magnesium.

Chromium: balancing energy levels

What it does

Chromium, along with B3, forms part of glucose tolerance factor (GTF), which is essential for balancing energy levels and helps to normalise hunger and reduce cravings – all key in pregnancy. It also improves lifespan, stimulates liver formation of important fats, helps protect DNA and RNA (our cells' genetic blueprint – particularly essential as your baby's cells proliferate), and is essential for heart function.

How much do I need?

The ideal daily intake is 50mcg, of which around 20mcg will need to be supplemented.

Best food sources: brewers yeast, wholemeal bread, rye bread, potatoes, wheatgerm, green peppers, eggs, chicken, apples, butter, parsnips, cornmeal, lamb chops, Swiss cheese.

Best supplement: chromium polynicotinate.

Iodine: key for brain development

What it does

When you're pregnant, your iodine requirements increase to help maintain your thyroid hormones, which are crucial for healthy development of your baby's brain and nervous system. A deficiency can lead to 'hypothyroidism' in your baby, which can cause mental retardation, deaf-mutism and spasticity.[6] A study carried out at Dundee University found that 40 per cent of women take less than half the recommended daily dose of iodine, and a deficiency could reduce the intelligence of their children.

How much do I need?

The ideal daily intake is 150mcg, of which around 50mcg will need to be supplemented.

Best food sources: haddock, mackerel, cod, yoghurt, pilchards, plaice, cheddar cheese, chicken.

Best supplement: most multi formulas designed for pregnant women include iodine, and if you eat fish, you'll get plenty from your diet.

Iron: preventing anaemia

Iron deficiency is very common in pregnancy. As many as 32 per cent of pregnant women may show mild iron deficiency anaemia, with symptoms of lethargy, pale skin and a sore tongue.

What it does

Iron is needed to make a protein in the blood called haemoglobin, which carries oxygen to every cell in the body. As blood volume increases during pregnancy, iron demand increases. Iron is also vital for energy production.

How much do I need?

The RDA for iron is 30mg but rarely more than 25mg is needed. However, pregnant women are often prescribed as much as 140mg. Except in cases where there has been excessive blood loss, such as an injury, this is far too much and interferes with the absorption of other minerals, especially zinc. During pregnancy 25mg is quite enough.

Best food sources: pumpkin seeds, parsley, almonds, dried prunes, cashews, raisins, Brazil nuts, walnuts, dates, pork, cooked dried beans, sesame seeds, pecans.

Best supplement: amino acid chelated iron is three times more absorbable than iron sulphate or oxide. Also good is iron citrate. Iron absorption is considerably enhanced by vitamin C so eating vitamin-C-rich foods helps – for example, having a glass of orange juice with your boiled egg can increase iron absorption fourfold.

Magnesium: for bones, heart and nervous system

Magnesium works with calcium and vitamin D to form your baby's bones and teeth. It's also key for the development of heart muscles and the nervous system. In you, it promotes healthy muscles by helping them to relax, so is important for labour cramps. Magnesium is also essential for energy production.

How much do I need?

The ideal daily intake for a pregnant woman is around 600mcg, of which around 300mcg will need to be supplemented.

Best food sources: wheatgerm, almonds, cashews, brewers yeast, buckwheat flour, Brazil nuts, peanuts, pecan nuts, cooked beans, garlic, raisins, green peas, potato skin, crab.

Best supplement: amino acid chelate or citrate is twice as well absorbed as magnesium carbonate or sulphate. It needs balancing with calcium and this should be the case in a multivitamin and mineral formula. However, if a multi formula doesn't give you enough (and it probably won't), we advise you take extra calcium and magnesium at a ratio of two parts calcium to one part magnesium.

Manganese: keeping you balanced

What it does

Manganese helps to form healthy bones, cartilage, tissues and nerves as well as promoting healthy DNA and RNA (our genetic blueprint), so is an essential mineral to have during pregnancy. It's also important for insulin production (the hormone that transports glucose from your blood to body cells, where energy is made) as well as brain function and also reduces cell damage.

How much do I need?

This mineral is often lacking in food – eating rich sources will provide around 3mg, but we recommend a daily intake of 5mg, so be sure to supplement 2mg.

Best food sources: watercress, pineapple, okra, endive, blackberries, raspberries, lettuce, grapes, lima beans, strawberries, oats, beetroot, celery.

Best supplement: amino acid chelate, manganese citrate or gluconate are the best sources. Take as part of a multi formula.

Selenium: boosting immunity

What it does

Selenium is an antioxidant so helps to protect against free radicals (toxic by-products of biochemical reactions in our bodies) and cancer-causing substances, which can interfere with your baby's development. It also reduces inflammation, stimulates your immune system to fight infections and promotes a healthy heart.

How much do I need?

An optimal diet should provide 20–25mcg, so supplement 40mcg to get the optimal daily intake of 60mcg.

Best food sources: molasses, mushrooms, herring, cottage cheese, cabbage, beef liver,* courgettes, cod, chicken.

Best supplement: selenomethionine, selenocysteine, but again you should get this in a good multivitamin or antioxidant supplement.

Zinc: for bigger, healthier babies

What it does

Of all the nutrients, zinc probably has the biggest role to play in reproduction. It's needed for hormone balance, development of sperm and egg, successful fertilisation and for all areas of your baby's growth. It

* See page 120 re. caution in eating liver during pregnancy

promotes a healthy nervous system and brain in both you and your baby, aids bone and teeth formation, helps hair to 'bloom' and is essential for constant energy. Research has shown that babies born to mothers who supplemented 25mg of zinc from the nineteenth week of pregnancy had a greater birth weight and head circumference.[7]

How much do I need?

A pregnant woman needs at least 20mg a day and frequently gets less than half of this from her diet. There are more grounds for supplementing zinc in pregnancy than any other mineral.

Best food sources: ginger root, lamb chops, pecans, dry split peas, haddock, green peas, shrimps, turnips, Brazil nuts, egg yolk, wholewheat grain, rye, oats, peanuts, almonds.

Best supplement: amino acid chelate, zinc citrate and picolinate are better than zinc sulphate or oxide. But again, you should get all you need in a good multi or antioxidant formula.

Best food sources

Foods vary widely in their nutrient content. You are most likely to get more vitamins and minerals in your food by:

- buying fresh, organic produce
- buying wholefoods (e.g. brown rice, beans, lentils) rather than refined or 'white' food (white bread, white pasta, etc.)
- choosing whole fruits and vegetables, and chopping or slicing just before eating
- eating fruit raw, and vegetables raw or lightly steamed, rather than overcooked or fried.

In summary, to ensure you get a good balance of all the essential vitamins and minerals you and your baby need:

- **Eat** at least three pieces of fresh fruit a day.

- **Have** a salad as a major part of one meal each day.

- **Eat** a multi-coloured variety of vegetables to get the best balance of nutrients (at least three portions a day).

- **Eat** wholefoods rather than refined or processed food full of artificial chemicals.

- **Eat** as much food as raw as possible. Prepare foods raw and heat to serve. When cooking, steam foods and fry as little as possible.

- **Wherever** possible, buy organic food and eat it quickly. If not possible, peel or throw away outer leaves and wash to reduce pesticide residues.

- **Supplement** your diet with a good multivitamin and mineral formula, plus extra nutrients as needed. When taking supplements make sure that natural sources of vitamins are used, which provide the full complement of other synergistic nutrients.

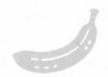

꩜

CHAPTER ELEVEN

The Better Pregnancy Diet

I N THE PREVIOUS two chapters, we've covered the specific nutrients you need to get from your diet to increase your chances of a healthy pregnancy with a super-healthy baby at the end. By now, you're probably getting a feel for the sort of food you should be eating. So let's translate this into actual meals and look at a typical menu plan over three days. Unless otherwise stated, the recipes serve one but quantities can easily be increased to cater for two or more.

DAY 1

Breakfast **Berry Booster**

> A delicious blend of a tub of natural yoghurt (cow, goat, sheep or soya), 2 handfuls of mixed berries (e.g. strawberries, blueberries, raspberries, blackcurrants), 1 tablespoon of wheatgerm or oatbran and 2 heaped tablespoons of freshly ground seeds (half flax, half pumpkin, sesame and sunflower, whizzed up in a coffee grinder).

Lunch **Red Cabbage and Mixed Vegetable Salad**

A colourful combination of chopped red cabbage and broccoli (½ cup each), 2 grated carrots, 2 sliced celery sticks, 2 chopped spring onions and ½ pack of smoked or marinated tofu, tossed in a cold-pressed seed oil and lemon juice dressing, sprinkled with fresh black pepper. Serve with rye or corn bread.

Supper **Roasted Vegetables with Pesto-crusted Chicken or Fish**

Add a pesto-coated organic chicken breast or fish fillet (organic salmon or cod works well) to a baking tray of part-roasted vegetables (e.g. new potatoes, cherry tomatoes, courgettes, onions, garlic, red and yellow peppers) and cook for a further 10–20 minutes. Season with salt and freshly ground pepper before serving.

Raspberry Sorbet

Liquidise frozen raspberries and bananas to a smooth purée.

Snacks Throughout the day, 3 pieces of seasonal fruit including an apple eaten with a large chunk of cheddar cheese or a handful of almonds.

Drinks Herb teas, Barleycup or dandelion coffee (available from healthfood shops), sparking mineral water and/or fresh juices diluted with water.

DAY 2

Breakfast **Simple fruit muesli**

Mix together 1 cup of porridge oats with 1 cup of chopped mixed fruit (e.g. apple, banana, mango, plums, apricots), 1 cup of cow, goat, soya or rice milk or natural yoghurt, 2 heaped tablespoons of ground seeds (as Day 1), and chopped almonds and hazelnuts.

Lunch **Spicy lentil and watercress soup (serves 2)**

A thick, nourishing combination of red split lentils (50g), cooked with a chopped onion and carrot in 1 pint of vegetable stock seasoned with a bay leaf and a good pinch of mild curry powder, thyme, celery salt and freshly ground black pepper. After 30 minutes, add 3 large handfuls of watercress and blend. Serve with wholemeal pitta bread and hummus.

Supper **Haddock poached in a parsley and lemon tofu sauce (serves 2)**

Blend ½ block of silken tofu with 1 small crushed clove of garlic, the juice of ½ lemon, some chopped parsley and salt and pepper. Add to a pan with 2 haddock fillets and slowly simmer so that the fish poaches (this will take about 15 minutes, but keep checking). Serve with steamed broccoli or other green vegetables and brown rice.

Dried fruit compote

Cover a mixture of dried fruit (e.g. prunes, figs, apricots, raisins, cherries) in boiling water, leave for 2 hours, then drain and simmer in a little water for 5 minutes. Stir in the juice and zest of an orange and serve with live natural yoghurt.

Snacks   Two pieces of fresh fruit or chopped vegetable sticks (e.g. carrots or celery) with a handful of pumpkin and sunflower seeds, and 2 oatcakes with cashew nut butter.

Drinks   As Day 1

DAY 3

Breakfast **Fruit milkshake**

A delicious creamy purée of fruit (try peaches, strawberries, banana, fresh dates or mango), ground seeds (as Day 1), vanilla essence and desiccated coconut, cow, goat or soya milk and ice.
A boiled free-range egg with wholemeal toast.

Lunch   **Filled jacket potato with fennel and tomato salad**

See page 116 for potato filling ideas. To make the salad, finely chop a bulb of fennel lengthways and mix with sliced tomatoes, a tablespoon of cold-pressed seed oil and lemon juice, then season with freshly ground pepper.

Supper   **Chickpea and apricot tagine (serves 2)**

To a basic tomato sauce (i.e. a tin of chopped tomatoes added to a chopped onion and chopped garlic clove softened in olive oil), stir in ½ a finely chopped red chilli and 1 pinch of ground cumin and simmer for 30–40 minutes. Add 1 handful of chopped dried apricots, 1 tin of chickpeas and 3 handfuls of chopped mixed vegetables (e.g. sugar snap peas, courgettes and baby corn) and cook for a further 10 minutes. Then stir in a handful of fresh chopped coriander and serve with couscous, quinoa or brown rice.

Apricot whisk (serves 2)

Purée a handful of apricots (fresh or dried) with ½ cup of low-fat curd cheese lightened with 2 whisked egg whites.

Snacks   A piece of fresh fruit such as an apple, a handful of almonds and carrot sticks with hummus.

Drinks   As Day 1

The dishes featured are quick and easy to prepare and can be adapted to suit your individual taste. Many are taken from the *Optimum Nutrition Cookbook* (by Patrick Holford and Judy Ridgway), so if you need more inspiration we suggest you refer to this book.

Other quick and easy meal ideas

Baked potato and sweet potato filling ideas:

- hummus (make your own or buy in the deli section of your supermarket) and roasted red peppers
- ratatouille or baked beans topped with grated cheddar cheese
- cottage cheese with chives or spring onion, mixed with chopped red or yellow peppers, cucumber or prawns
- roasted vegetables and pesto
- tinned or smoked salmon mixed with cottage cheese or crème fraîche
- cannelini or butter beans mashed with anchovy fillets and black olives, with lemon juice and black pepper
- steamed leeks, broccoli or cauliflower florets mixed with béchamel sauce with cheese
- hard-boiled egg chopped and mixed with cottage cheese or crème fraîche and chopped parsley

- guacamole (with mashed avocado, a mashed tomato, chopped garlic and a touch of chilli sauce and lemon juice).

Delicious salads and light meals (perfect for a packed lunch):

A simple salad of mixed leaves and chopped raw vegetables can become a nutritious and delicious meal in moments if you keep your fridge stocked with deli delights such as artichoke hearts, sun-blushed tomatoes, olives, hard-boiled eggs, peppers, bottled sweet baby peppers, anchovies, smoked fish and slices of lean white meat. Here are some ideas to 'theme' your salad:

- Smoked organic trout fillet (a delicious alternative to smoked salmon that is packed with Omega 3 essential fats) with flageolet beans or lightly steamed broad beans mixed with lemon juice and black pepper.

- Hot organic trout or salmon, or smoked organic mackerel, flaked through wholegrains such as quinoa, brown rice, millet or cous cous, with chopped raw vegetables. Season with lemon juice, balsamic vinegar, black pepper and chopped fresh herbs.

- Tofu chunks (marinated in tamari or soy sauce, ginger, garlic and sesame oil and brown rice syrup), stir-fried for 7 minutes or until fairly crisp. Toss through wholegrains as above, or stir into buckwheat noodles with finely sliced cucumber and seaweed (packets of dried varieties can be found in the Oriental section of supermarkets). Sprinkle with sesame seeds and serve warm or chilled.

- Mixed bean salad with peppers, cherry tomatoes, red onion, bottled sweet baby peppers and chopped hard-boiled egg, with a tomato and basil dressing.

- Chickpeas dressed with paprika, lemon juice, black pepper and a sprinkle of sea salt or Solo low sodium salt and parsley, with quinoa.

- Warm potato salad with sundried tomatoes and diced avocado with a dressing made from olive oil, paprika, chillies and crushed garlic.

- Taboulleh of cous cous, bulgar wheat, millet or quinoa with chopped cherry tomatoes, spring onions, cucumber, parsley, mint, olive oil, lemon juice and seasoning.

- Whole radishes, crumbled feta cheese, broad beans and alfalfa sprouts.

- Blueberries and apricots on green leaves such as lamb's leaf or spinach, with feta cheese crumbled over the top.

Foods to beware

There are certain foods we may normally eat without any problem but that for pregnant women carry a slight risk of infection. Although this risk is very small (for example, you have a 1 in 29,000 chance of getting listeria from eating soft cheese), food poisoning and parasites can have a serious impact on your developing baby. So it's wise to avoid some foods and take more care while preparing others when you're pregnant and breast feeding.

- **Paté and soft or blue cheeses** such as Brie, Camembert, Stilton, Roquefort, Boursin and soft goat or sheep cheeses can be contaminated with listeria, as can soft-whip ice creams and unpasteurised milk (although the risk of unpasteurised cheeses such as Parmesan and Gruyère is so minor they're OK to eat). Hard pasteurised cheese such as cheddar and Nanny's goat cheddar or cottage cheese are safer bets.

- **Raw eggs and poultry** can harbour salmonella – in fact it's estimated that as much as 33 per cent of fresh and 41 per cent of frozen chickens are infected[8] – so make sure you cook both thoroughly (for eggs, this means until both white and yolk turn solid) and avoid buying chilled pre-cooked chicken or having foods made with raw eggs such as fresh mayonnaise or chocolate mousse.

- **Raw shellfish and sushi**, unless really fresh, can cause serious food poisoning so are best avoided. Sushi can also contain parasites if not prepared properly. Because of high levels of mercury contamination, it's advisable to avoid fish such as shark, swordfish and marlin, and limit tuna to just once a week, if at all.

- **Green or sprouting potatoes** contain poisonous substances called alpha-solanine and alpha-chaconine, which are linked to spina bifida. So be sure you don't eat sprouted potatoes and cut away any green areas before cooking.

- **Peanuts** can cause serious allergic reactions and the number of children affected has dramatically increased in recent years. For this reason, some health professionals suggest pregnant women avoid them, but we feel this is unnecessary unless you already have a child with allergies to peanuts or there's a strong family history of allergies. However, choose organic peanuts, as these have been found to contain fewer aflatoxins, a toxic mould.

- **Wash fruit and vegetables** thoroughly to remove any traces of soil or bacteria. Even ready-prepared salads can be contaminated, so wash these too.

- **Cook meat** properly to kill off any bacteria and keep uncooked meat away from any cooked foods in your fridge to avoid cross-contamination. Be sure to wash your hands and utensils thoroughly after preparing meat and don't use the same chopping board as you do for vegetables or bread.

A few more cautions

- **Coffee and caffeine-containing drinks**, as explored in Part One, can have a negative impact on fertility. But once you're pregnant, many British doctors claim that a few cups a day is OK, although anything more may increase the risk of miscarriage. However, caffeine crosses the placenta and affects the baby in the same way as it affects the mother – i.e. it increases heart and breathing rate and alters neuro-behaviour. As a growing baby is not yet developed, the effects are likely to be more profound. A baby is also less able to detoxify caffeine and it's estimated to stay in their bloodstream for up to 100 hours. In the US, the Food and Drug Administration (FDA) advises pregnant women to avoid caffeine-containing foods and drugs (and this includes colas) completely.[9] We advise the same. Decaffeinated coffee still contains two other stimulants (theobromine and theophylline) and can be more toxic due to the chemicals used to remove the caffeine, but if you want to enjoy the occasional cup, buy an organic variety where the caffeine is removed via the safer 'Swiss water process' (in the UK, Taylors coffee is decaffeinated this way).

- **Alcohol** is also toxic and not safe for your developing baby at any level. As discussed, only a few glasses of wine a week can increase risk of miscarriage and cause damage to your baby's brain and nervous system (see chapter 4 for more on this). So, again, we advise you don't drink alcohol at all while pregnant or breast feeding.

- **Liver** is often warned against during pregnancy because of its high vitamin A content. However, as discussed in chapter 5, you need vitamin A when you're pregnant. So while we don't advise you stop eating it altogether, we do suggest you limit your consumption to a small portion every other week and eat only organic, as non-organic will be contaminated with growth hormones, steroids and antibiotics used in conventional farming (the liver being the place all these get stored). However, if you do continue to eat liver make sure any supplements you take don't have any extra animal-derived vitamin A (retinol) but only the vegetable source (betacarotene). This will especially apply to cod liver oil, a very rich source of retinol. If you don't eat liver make sure your multivitamin provides at least 1,000mcg of retinol.

How much extra do I need to eat?

While every calorie you eat needs to be nutrient-rich to nourish both you and your baby throughout your pregnancy, it's not necessary to eat for two. In fact, you don't actually need to eat any more until the last three months, and even then it's only an extra 200 calories (the equivalent of an apple and 1 oz/28g of cheddar cheese). The daily calorie guide for the 'average' woman is 2,000 calories, increasing to 2,200 calories in months seven, eight and nine of pregnancy. Then, after you give birth, you'll need an extra 500 calories a day while you're breast feeding.

Fuel for a successful labour

Two weeks before your due date, stock up on plenty of complex carbohydrates (i.e. wholegrains and vegetables) as these are the main energy source for the body. You may also want to take a GLA (an essential fat) supplement – 500mg of evening primrose or blackcurrant seed oil will help you make substances called prostaglandins that prepare your cervix for the birth. Raspberry leaf tea also helps to relax and tone the uterus – so drink several cups a day (you can buy it from health-food shops). Although thankfully rare now, some hospitals still starve women in labour just in case there's a need for an anaesthetic. Yet in terms of energy requirements, labour can be compared to a marathon run. After all the good work you have done to create a healthy baby, the last thing you want is to run out of energy and have a prolonged labour that may result in Caesarean delivery and increase your baby's risks of birth-related trauma. If your hospital allows you to eat and drink, we recommend that you drink diluted grape juice, which supplies a very healthy and readily available source of fruit sugar that should help keep up your energy levels. Caffeinated tea, with or without sugar, will not give you stable energy levels, so avoid this if offered. And if you feel hungry, snack on seeds and nuts, oatcakes with nut butter and sticks of carrots or celery.

CHAPTER TWELVE

∾

Why Supplements are Essential

I F YOUR DOCTOR or midwife tells you that you don't need supplements, find a new one. They may even say 'as long as you eat a
well-balanced diet you'll get all the nutrients you need'. This is
the biggest lie in nutrition today. Every survey conducted in Britain
since the 1980s shows that even those who said that they ate a balanced diet fail to eat anything like the European or American recommended daily allowances (RDAs) of vitamins and minerals. And
as we've seen already (page 98), these RDAs aren't even designed to
ensure optimal health, rather to prevent severe nutritional deficiency
diseases such as scurvy.

No doubt you will have been told to supplement folic acid. But why
not any other essential nutrients for which there is equally good evidence of a shortfall, and an additional benefit during pregnancy? Zinc
is an example of another vital nutrient for your baby. So strong is the
link, that your baby's size and head circumference at birth is predictable just by knowing the level of zinc in the placenta! The average
intake of zinc is 7.6mg, while the EU RDA is 15mg. In the US the recommendation during pregnancy is 20mg. That's a big shortfall! By the
way, we agree with the Americans on this one.

The reason why folic acid is recommended is that the average
intake of folic acid is 250mcg. The ideal during pregnancy is probably

closer to 600mcg. The UK Department of Health recommends that a woman wishing to get pregnant, or who is actually pregnant, supplement 400mcg. This is good, but probably not enough for many people. Folic acid, along with B12 and B6, are essential for proper growth of the baby. We recommend supplementing all of these.

Why, you may ask, when food is so abundant in our society, are we not getting the nutrients we need? First, we never did. The idea that we (humanity) were dropped into a garden of Eden, complete with 'optimum nutrition', doesn't match the facts. All species compete for nutrients. Those that get good at exploiting particular environments become dominant, like us. Others, like the dodo, become extinct. Only now has humanity become so adept at exploiting the environment and at the same time has the knowledge about nutrition even to have the choice of being optimally nourished. We are certainly lucky in that respect, so let's take advantage of it and reap the rewards in better health.

To do this, however, you need to be canny to get what you need. Over-farmed soils are mineral depleted and refining or processing food diminishes nutrients (for example, white flour, rice and sugar have 77 per cent less zinc, chromium and manganese than brown), as does cooking. Unless you're fortunate, most food you buy isn't locally grown and has often travelled hundreds (or even thousands) of miles to your supermarket shelf – a factor that further depletes nutrient content. For these reasons – plus the length of time we store foods – there's a staggering variation in the nutrient content in fruit and vegetables. For example, an orange may provide from zero to 180mg of vitamin C, the average being around 60mg. Yes, some supermarket oranges contain no vitamin C! Or a large (100g) carrot can provide from 21mcg to 5,000mcg of vitamin A. This is partly due to the long time it takes to get a carrot from the field to your mouth, but it's largely due to intensive farming practices using fertilisers that mean big, cheap carrots or oranges, regardless of their quality. That's why buying fresh organic food, not pre-chopped, and eating it quickly once you've chopped it up, gives you more nutrients from your food.

So while the Better Pregnancy Diet encourages you to eat nutrient-rich and preferably organic food, it's still necessary to supplement with extra vitamins and minerals to guarantee you get optimum levels to help both you and your developing baby achieve the best health possible. Supplements do have to guarantee what they contain. Foods don't. Supplementation is especially important in pregnancy as your nutrient needs are even greater than usual – your requirements for folic acid and other B vitamins, vitamin C, calcium, zinc and magnesium, for example, increase by 30 to 100 per cent.

Studies show that pregnant women who supplement their diet with a multivitamin reduce the risk of having a baby with a birth defect by 30–35 per cent.[10] Taking supplements also reduces the risk of having a premature or low birth-weight baby – in one study in the US, city-dwelling women on low incomes (i.e. those more likely to have a nutrient-deficient diet) halved their risk by taking a multivitamin and mineral supplement for the first six months of pregnancy.[11]

Before we look at which supplements you should be taking, let's first determine the 'Optimum Level' of each essential vitamin and mineral you should be getting every day. Of course, this depends on your individual needs, which is why we recommend seeing a nutritional therapist who can work this out for you (see Resources for details). However the Optimum Levels, shown in the first column of the table opposite, are good averages based on our experience and current nutritional research.

The 'Optimum Dietary Intake' column shows the levels that an optimum diet, as outlined in chapters 9, 10 and 11, can supply. This is roughly what you should achieve if you follow our recommendations.

The next column, 'Minimum Supplemental Level', represents the difference, in other words what you need to supplement to reach the Optimum Levels, given that you are eating an optimal diet. Finally, the last column gives the EU RDAs for your interest – you will see how far below these often are for achieving what we consider the best health possible. That's why we nickname them the 'Ridiculous Dietary Arbitraries'!

Nutrient	Optimum level	Optimum dietary intake	Minimum supplemental level during pregnancy	RDA
Vitamins				
A (retinol)	1,500mcg	750mcg	750mcg*	(800mcg)
A (beta-carotene)	1,500mcg	750mcg	750mcg	(2.2mcg)
D	120mcg	60mcg	60mcg	(10–20mcg)
E	270mg	13mg	255mg	(3–4mg)
C	1,500mg	200mg	1,300mg	(70mg)
B1 (thiamine)	25mg	2mg	23mg	(1.5mg)
B2 (riboflavin)	25mg	3 mg	22mg	(1.6mg)
B3 (niacin)	50mg	25mg	25mg	(17mg)
B5 (pantothenic acid)	50mg	30mg	20mg	(–)
B6 (pyridoxine)	60mg	10mg	50mg*	(2.2mg)
B12	60mcg	10mcg	50mcg	(2.2mcg)
Folic Acid	800mcg	200mcg	600mcg	(400mcg)
Biotin	100mcg	50mcg	50mcg	(400mcg)
Minerals				
Calcium	1,200mg	600mg	600mg	(1,200mg)
Copper	50mcg	50mcg	–	(2.2mcg)
Magnesium	600mg	300mg	300mg	(320mg)
Iron	25mg	15mg	10mg	(30mg)
Zinc	20mg	10mg	10mg	(15mg)
Manganese	5mg	3mg	2mg	(1.8mg)
Chromium	50mcg	30mcg	20mcg	(25mcg)
Selenium	60mcg	20mcg	40mcg	(65mcg)
Iodine	150mcg	100mcg	50mcg	(175mcg)

* A note on safety: the levels of nutrients included in different supplement formulas varies enormously, so use this as a rough guide. Any of the 'Minimum Supplementation Levels' are still perfectly safe at double the quantities given. A word of caution on two nutrients, however. Don't supplement more than 3,000mcg (10,000iu) of the retinol form of vitamin A (see page 99 for more on this), and don't supplement more than 100mg of B6, as higher doses may suppress your milk production when you start breast feeding.

Your supplement programme for a healthy pregnancy

If trying to get your head around this list makes you want to close the book in despair, wait! Many nutrient formulas do the hard work for you by combining all the necessary vitamins and minerals into a few single supplements. Although it would be ideal to seek expert help to formulate your individual supplementary needs preconceptually and during pregnancy, there are also plenty of ready-made supplements designed specifically for pregnant women if you decide not to do this. See the Resources section for a list of good supplement suppliers and how to find a nutritional therapist.

To cover all the basics, our recommendation is to take three supplements:

* An optimum nutrition or pregnancy multivitamin and mineral formula (good ones normally say 'take two a day' – you just can't get enough in one tablet).

* 1,000–2,000mg of extra vitamin C.

* An essential fat formula providing 400mg EPA, 200mg of DHA and 200mg of GLA (see chapter 8 for more about essential fats).

Optional:

* A combined calcium and magnesium supplement if you can't find a multivitamin/mineral that includes the levels we recommend. Aim to get two parts calcium to one part magnesium, for example 400mg of calcium and 200mg of magnesium.

* An antioxidant if you are an older mother (i.e. over thirty), live in a polluted environment, are at risk of developing pre-eclampsia or are under a lot of stress. A good formula should provide extra beta-carotene, vitamin E, selenium and zinc, and other beneficial antioxidants such as reduced glutathione, N-acetyl Cysteine, co-enzyme Q10 and alpha-lipoic acid.

When and how to take supplements:

- Take your multi (and antioxidant and calcium/magnesium if applicable) with breakfast and, if necessary, again at lunch and dinner (i.e. if two or three are recommended to meet your daily intake).

- Likewise, vitamin C (i.e. split into 500mg doses).

- Take essential fats with a meal that contains some fat to aid absorption.

- Take all these supplements with food.

By the way, you may find your urine becomes yellower. This is normal. Just drink more water and know that, like water, the body is designed to excrete essential nutrients. It's what they do in between that counts.

Family history of allergies?

Each of us is born with a sterile gut, but by the time we reach adulthood, about 2kg (5lb) of bacteria has taken up residence. The majority of this bacteria is 'friendly' in that it helps to break down our food, make certain B vitamins and vitamin K and prevent any nasty bacteria (i.e. bugs that cause food poisoning) from taking up residence. However, the balance between friendly and harmful bacteria can sometimes shift in the wrong direction if you have too many antibiotics, steroid drugs or artificial hormones (including the Pill), eat a diet high in refined carbohydrates or are under long-term stress. This can cause a variety of digestive problems and can also lead to allergies and related conditions such as asthma and eczema. If you have a family history of any of these, you can help prevent passing them on to your baby by ensuring your gut bacteria is healthy. Research has shown that supplementing your diet with a probiotic – a good guy version of an antibiotic, which replenishes stores of good bacteria – can reduce the likelihood of allergies in your baby by

50 per cent. Doing this can also help to prevent your baby inheriting eczema or asthma.[12] So our advice, if this applies to you, is to take a probiotic supplement (containing both lactobacillus and acidophilus strains) daily throughout your pregnancy and continue while breast feeding. See the Resources section for suppliers.

❦

CHAPTER THIRTEEN

Preventing Problems: from Anaemia to Weight Gain

I F YOU FOLLOW the Better Pregnancy Diet and Supplement Plan, you should not only be in great shape, you will also minimise your chances of suffering any of the problems that can occur during pregnancy. By knowing what these are and taking simple precautionary measures, you can often prevent them happening, or at least alleviate the symptoms. Here are some of the more common problems you might encounter.

Anaemia

Mild anaemia may occur in as many as one in three pregnant women. The symptoms include pallor, tiredness, a sore tongue and a feeling almost as if there's a weight on your shoulders. It's usually the result of a low level of iron in the blood protein haemoglobin, although B12, folic acid, manganese and B6 deficiency can also result in anaemia. Supplementing 20mg of iron in the ferrous, not ferric, form (for example, ferrous sulphate) should alleviate this problem – if you're already taking a multivitamin and mineral formula, you'll only need to take an extra 10mg or so. Occasionally, as much as 40mg may be required but as you'll be tested throughout your pregnancy, your doctor should prescribe this for you if necessary. However, don't take any more than this as it can interfere with the absorption of other essential minerals such as zinc. Studies have also shown that higher doses don't result in increased levels of iron in the blood, as measured by your haemoglobin count. But eating iron-rich foods (see page 107) will further boost levels, as will having vitamin-C-rich foods at the same time, which enhance iron absorption by up to twice as much. So enjoy a glass or fresh orange juice with a boiled egg, or have some seeds or nuts with a piece of fruit.

Backache

The tendons supporting your back become softer in pregnancy due to increased levels of the hormone progesterone. As your baby grows, your centre of gravity is pushed further forwards and, to compensate, many women push their shoulders back and their tummies out, putting strain on their backs. That's why it's particularly important to maintain good posture. Imagine you are held up by a string attached to the top of your head, and keep your shoulders relaxed. When you are sitting don't slouch, and if you feel you need some support for the lower back, put a cushion between you and the back of the chair. Try to avoid lifting heavy objects. When you do lift don't do it by bending over and straining your back muscles. Instead, bend your knees and keep your back straight, taking the weight with your thigh muscles.

Constipation

Many people imagine their abdominal organs – stomach, liver, pancreas, bladder and intestines – live in spacious surroundings. Actually, they are closely packed together. The arrival of a baby plus placenta, enlarged uterus and fluid, is a very tight fit and results in less room for the intestines, stomach and bladder to expand. For many women this means a greater chance of constipation, since the faecal matter in the large intestine is more compressed and the muscles have less room to keep the contents moving along. The answer is not to take laxatives, but to make sure your diet is especially high in fluids and fibre and low in mucus-forming foods. Dairy products, eggs and meat are especially mucus forming and tend to make faecal matter more compacted and harder to pass along. On the other hand, fruits, vegetables, grains, lentils and beans are high in fibre and this fibre absorbs fluid, making the resulting faecal matter light and bulky and easier to pass. It is a good idea to drink at least 1.5 litres (about 2.5 pints) of filtered or bottled water a day, either as it is or as diluted fruit juice. (By the way, drinking more water will in no way encourage fluid retention.) Stirring a dessertspoon of flaxseeds into a glass of water before bed, then drinking the gel-like solution down in the morning, followed by another glass of water, will also help to loosen things up.

Cravings

Low zinc levels are associated with the abnormal cravings a pregnant woman often experiences in early pregnancy. In addition, replenishing low iron levels in the body has been successfully used to control abnormal cravings that some women experience for strange, and sometimes harmful, substances such as chalk or coal. Following the Better Pregnancy Diet and Supplement Plan should replenish these, but if they persist, see a nutritional therapist who can test your mineral levels (see the Resources section at the back of this book).

Depression

About 10 per cent of pregnant women – 13 per cent to 15 per cent among new mothers – develop depression severe enough to interfere with their functioning. But you can do a lot to reduce your risk by being optimally nourished. Two main players in pregnancy-related depression are zinc and essential fats.

In a study of 11,721 British women, researchers found that those who consumed greater amounts of seafood (a rich source of both essential fats and zinc) during the last three months of their pregnancy were less likely to show signs of major depression before and for up to eight months after the birth. Women with the highest intakes of Omega 3, who consumed fish two or three times a week, were half as likely to suffer from depression as women with the lowest intakes.[13] By following the Better Pregnancy Diet and Supplement Plan, your intake of zinc and essential fats should be optimal, so if you feel low, check you're getting what you should (see pages 75–85 and 109) and also that your blood sugar is balanced (see page 93). For more on post-natal depression, see page 169.

Gestational diabetes

Gestational diabetes is an extreme form of poor blood glucose control (see page 10), where the body is unable to maintain a constant energy level. It usually occurs during the second half of pregnancy and disappears after birth, but it can be an early warning sign of the mother developing diabetes later in life. Your baby may be bigger, increasing the chances of Caesarean delivery, and the baby also has a greater risk of developing diabetes. This condition affects up to 3 in every 100 women and manifests as a whole host of symptoms including fatigue, poor concentration, irritability, nervousness, depression, excessive thirst, sweating, headaches and digestive problems. If you are diagnosed with gestational diabetes, the diet outlined in this book will help you control it. In particular:

- Eat complex carbohydrates that release their energy slowly (i.e. rye bread, oats, brown rice, vegetables) and avoid refined carbohydrates (i.e. white bread, biscuits, cakes) and any foods with added sugar.

- Balance meals and snacks with protein – so eat some seeds and yoghurt with your breakfast cereal or have a boiled egg, make sure main meals include some lean meat, fish, pulses or dairy products, and balance snacks, so have an apple with ten almonds, hummus and carrot or celery sticks or nut butter on oatcakes, for example.

- Make sure you include lots of fibre in your diet as this slows down the release of glucose into your blood. Eating plenty of wholegrains will help, as will lots of vegetables and fruit (but balance fruit with protein, as above).

- Take a multivitamin and mineral to boost nutrient levels, but supplement extra chromium and B3 specifically to help your body manage glucose. You can usually buy these combined in a 'Glucose Tolerance' formula – look for up to 200mcg of chromium and 25mg of B3. See the Resources section for suppliers.

Heartburn

In the last months of pregnancy it's common to experience some heartburn because of the pressure of an enlarged uterus on your stomach. There is no magical cure, other than to avoid the foods that trigger it, and to eat small amounts little and often rather than having big meals. You may find it helpful to sleep slightly propped up towards the end of pregnancy. But do avoid antacids as a remedy, as these commonly contain aluminium, which is toxic. A quarter of a teaspoonful of sodium bicarbonate dissolved in water and taken between meals can bring relief.

High blood pressure

Raised blood pressure commonly occurs in pregnancy and an optimum diet should help to control it. Evening primrose oil and calcium have both been used successfully to reduce it – see the section on pre-eclampsia for doses and other suggestions.

Leg cramps

Cramps are nearly always due to an imbalance of calcium and magnesium. These minerals, as well as sodium and potassium, are called electrolytes because they control the electrical balance that causes muscles to relax and contract. A cramp happens when muscles go into contraction. As a growing baby needs lots of magnesium and calcium to build its bones, pregnant women can often become deficient. So follow the Better Pregnancy Diet and Supplement Plan, eat lots of calcium and magnesium balanced foods such as green leafy vegetables, nuts and seeds and supplement 600mg calcium with 300mg of magnesium each day. Make sure you also get plenty of fluids, as dehydration can make cramps worse.

Morning (noon and night) sickness

During the first three months of pregnancy all the organs of your baby are completely formed. It is during this period – and, of course, before conception – that optimum nutrition is most important. Yet many women experience continual sickness at this time and don't feel like eating healthily. Misnamed 'morning' sickness, the most common signs and symptoms are nausea, usually worse on an empty stomach, and often triggered by the smells of certain foods or perfumes; vomiting after eating; aversions to some foods and cravings for others; a metallic taste in the mouth; a feeling of hunger even when feeling nauseous; and relief from nausea by eating.

Pregnancy sickness is one example of a condition that usually only manifests in women whose nutritional status is less than optimum. Probably caused by an increase in a hormone called human chorionic gonadotrophin (HCG), women with poor diets are particularly at risk.[14] HCG is produced by the developing placenta from the moment of conception and usually reaches its peak around nine to ten weeks after the last period, before declining by week fourteen to sixteen. In very undernourished mothers HCG may not be produced in sufficient quantities at all, which may explain why women who miscarry early on are less likely to experience any pregnancy sickness. Conversely, very well-nourished women appear to ride the storm of these hormonal changes with little or no symptoms of nausea at all.

Other possible explanations for nausea or sickness involve the body trying to eliminate toxins, and also difficulty maintaining blood sugar balance. The Better Pregnancy Diet and Supplement Plan reduces toxins and evens out blood sugar; it also provides sufficient levels of nutrients to balance hormones. But if you still suffer, try the following:

- Always eat breakfast, preferably containing some protein foods such as yoghurt or eggs.

- Eat small meals and frequent snacks of fruit and seeds.

- Avoid refined and sugary foods.

- Avoid high-fat junk food containing long lists of additives and preservatives.

- Decrease your intake of dried fruit or undiluted fruit juice, both of which provide concentrated sugar.

- Drink plenty of water between meals.

- Avoid or decrease your intake of coffee and tea.

- Take a multivitamin containing a good level of all the B vitamins and zinc.

- If sickness persists, take 50mg of vitamin B6 twice a day and 200–500mg of magnesium once a day until the sickness subsides.

- Ginger may help to relieve the sickness and settle your stomach – take either in capsules or as tea.

Pre-eclampsia

Pre-eclampsia (also called toxaemia) is a condition that only occurs after the fifth or sixth month of pregnancy and affects one in ten women pregnant for the first time. It is usually caused by a poorly functioning placenta and oxidative stress to the blood vessels. The first sign is raised blood pressure, which may be accompanied by slight swelling in the ankles. You'll have your blood pressure checked during your medical check-ups. If you do experience swelling in your ankles or have high blood pressure your doctor may want to do a urine test to check if you have protein in the urine. This is a sign of pre-eclampsia. Once the pregnancy is over the symptoms go away. However, if it progresses unchecked, pre-eclampsia can develop into eclampsia, a life-threatening condition where convulsive seizures can occur. It is for this reason that regular check-ups are very important since women with pre-eclampsia don't necessarily feel ill.

Developing pre-eclampsia is very unlikely if you are following our Better Pregnancy Diet and Supplement Plan. This is because people who eat more fruit and vegetables, and supplement vitamin B, C, E and essential fats, have a fraction of the risk.[15]

Stretchmarks

The skin on the abdomen does a remarkable stretching job in pregnancy, but if it expands beyond its elastic capacity, stretch marks can develop. Stretch marks on the stomach, thighs, breasts, hips or shoulder girdle are one of the signs of zinc deficiency, so eating zinc-rich foods, such as nuts, fish, peas and eggs, as well as ensuring you get 15mg of zinc in your daily supplement, is crucial. Vitamin C is also needed to make collagen, the intercellular glue; and vitamin E helps to keep skin supple. So make sure your diet provides plenty of these vitamins and again, supplement at the levels suggested (see chapter 10). Applying vitamin E oil (from a vitamin E capsule is best so it's not damaged) or cream is also helpful during the last weeks of pregnancy and after the birth to encourage the skin to contract. The skin flexibility also depends on essential fats, so make sure your intake of essential fats is optimal (see chapter 8).

Varicose veins

Varicose veins are fairly common during pregnancy. They develop because of restricted blood flow and also constipation. All the blood vessels in the feet and legs lead to one big vein in the groin, but if this is compressed by the baby or by a build-up of waste matter in the bowel, the blood must return along different routes. This can cause small veins on the surface of the legs to become enlarged. The result is prominent veins that may become varicose veins.

The secret of avoiding varicose veins is to keep your blood vessels in good shape and to minimise the restriction of blood flow. Vitamin C is needed to make collagen, which keeps the arteries supple. Vitamin B3 helps to dilate the blood vessels, while vitamin E and the essential fatty acid EPA thin the blood and help to transport oxygen. Regular exercise will also help to stimulate proper circulation.

Water retention

Hormonal changes during pregnancy can mean your body holds on to more sodium, and this increases the amount of fluid in your body. So cut down on salty foods (e.g. bacon, crisps, canned or processed foods) and boost your intake of potassium-rich foods, such as fruit and vegetables, which help to balance out excess sodium levels. Don't make the mistake of thinking that drinking water will make the problem worse – quite the reverse as it will help to 'flush' out your system, so aim to have 1.5 to 2 litres (2.5 to 3.5 pints) a day. Regular exercise will also help to boost lymphatic drainage (your internal cleansing system). And make sure you're not constipated (see page 130), as this will prevent toxins being eliminated and encourage water retention.

What about weight gain?

By the end of your pregnancy, your baby may weigh between 3.5 and 4kg (7.7 and 8.8lb), but you're likely to have gained around 12.5kg (28lb). Much of this is the placenta, fluid and increase in blood volume that supports the baby, but your body will also store more fat as an energy reserve while your baby is growing and in preparation for breast feeding.

As a general guide, you're likely to gain about 4kg (8lb) by the end of the first twenty weeks, and about a pound per week after that. However, each woman is different. If your weight gain is more, check you are not eating for two (you only need an extra 200 calories a day in the last three months) or filling up on empty calories (i.e. refined, sugary or processed foods) or not exercising enough. Giving birth can be like running a marathon, and you need to be fit. You could also be suffering from water retention (see earlier). If your weight gain is less than half this amount, it is important to check that you are eating enough. Since the more important measure is whether the baby is growing, measuring your waist is a better indication than your weight.

Birth-weight: why bigger is better

The size of your baby when you give birth is a strong indictor of his or her future health and intelligence – not just in the early stages of development, but throughout life. Professor David Barker from The Medical Research Council Epidemiology Unit at Southampton University has extensively researched the connection between birth-weight and disease in adulthood. He's been able to clearly show that babies weighing less than 2.5kg (5.5lb) (the official definition of a low birth-weight baby) are more inclined to develop heart disease, stroke, diabetes and other diseases in later life. Not only is a good birth-weight (between 3.5–4kg or 7.7–8.8lb) a key factor of future health; it also reduces your baby's chances of handicap or death. And the larger your baby is at birth, the more intelligent they are likely to be – in a study that followed 3,900 British men and women born in 1946, birth-weight was found to be significantly related to intellectual development and educational achievement in later life.[16] However, it's not necessarily the quantity of food you eat while pregnant, rather the quality that's key for a healthy birth-weight. In a study of women who'd had babies with low birth-weight, tests revealed they were deficient in forty-three out of forty-four nutrients measured.[17] So swap refined carbohydrates such as sweets, cakes, biscuits and white bread – which can actually increase both your and your baby's risk of developing diabetes – for nutrient-dense wholegrains, fruits, vegetables, good quality protein, nuts and seeds. Take regular exercise too, as this has also been shown to increases birth-weight.[18] Finally, if the thought of giving birth to a bigger baby makes you shudder, there's no need to grin and bear it. Babies that weigh more aren't necessarily any more painful or difficult to deliver than smaller ones – factors such as the shape of your pelvis, position of the baby and preparation for birth have far greater implications.

❧

CHAPTER FOURTEEN

Vital Energy Boosters

BEING PREGNANT MAKES extra demands on your energy – after all, you're making and carrying another human being around, albeit a small one. But while you'll undoubtedly feel a bit more tired than usual, if you were prone to fatigue before conceiving, being pregnant can be exhausting. The best way to boost your energy is by eating a nutrient-rich diet and balancing your blood sugar while eliminating foods that drain your body's resources. Taking time out to relax and doing some exercise will also increase your energy and vitality.

Avoid energy lows

As explained in chapter 9, the type of carbohydrate we eat determines how efficient we are at making energy. Carbohydrate is broken down into glucose, then transported via the blood to body cells, where it's burnt (or metabolised) to make energy. Any excess glucose is converted to glycogen (a short-term fuel stored mainly in the liver and muscle cells) or fat, our long-term energy reserve.

But if your main supply of carbohydrate releases its glucose too fast, for example because you eat refined and sugary foods, then you get a sudden rush of energy (or blood glucose high), which is quickly followed by an energy low.

Keeping your blood glucose balanced is probably the most important factor in maintaining stable energy levels and not gaining any excess weight – not just while you're pregnant, but also throughout your life. The level of glucose in your blood largely determines your appetite. When the level drops, you feel hungry. But if levels drop too low, you can experience a whole host of symptoms including fatigue, poor concentration, irritability, nervousness, depression, excessive thirst, sweating, headaches and digestive problems. An estimated three in every ten people have difficulty keeping their blood sugar level even, with sudden highs followed by deep lows. The result, over the years, is that they become increasingly lethargic and often overweight. On the other hand, if you can control your blood sugar levels the result is constant energy and no excess weight gain.

If you find you can't go for more than a few hours without eating and/or often crave sweet foods or stimulants (i.e. tea, coffee, chocolate, cola), then you can take positive steps to balance your energy better.

Avoid	Instead
Refined or white carbohydrates – white bread, white rice, cakes, biscuits, etc.	Eat wholegrain foods – wholemeal or rye bread, brown rice, oatcakes.
Sugary foods such as sweets or fizzy drinks.	Eat fresh fruit – especially apples, cherries, oranges, plums, grapes, pears, grapefruit.
Artificial sweeteners as these can be harmful to health.	Sweeten food with fruit or honey, or buy brown rice syrup (from healthfood shops).
Stimulants – tea, coffee, chocolate, cola, (alcohol and cigarettes).	Drink plenty of water and dilute fruit juices 50/50 with water.
Carbohydrate-only meals or snacks (i.e. pasta with tomato sauce, a banana on its own).	Balance carbohydrate with protein – so eat some fish with your salad, mix lentils with your rice, eat a handful of nuts, seeds or a piece of cheese with your fruit.

Skipping meals.   Aim to eat three meals a day with
                                   two snacks in between breakfast and
                                   lunch and lunch and supper.

Instant energy boosters

Balancing your blood sugar will greatly increase your energy. But if
you need an extra boost, here are some instant ways to energise yourself:

- Make a fresh juice – raw foods give you an energy lift. A juicer is a
  good investment and you can experiment with different combinations to find ones you like best. Try apple and/or orange with carrot;
  celery, spinach and beetroot; or apple, grape and berry (any sort –
  blueberry, raspberry, blackberry). Dilute fruit juices 50/50 with still
  or sparkling water to slow down the glucose release.

- Have a salad with some sprouted seeds – fresh, living foods give you
  lots more energy than dead, processed foods. You can buy alfalfa,
  lentil or bean sprouts from healthfood shops, or try sprouting your
  own (many healthfood shops sell kits with full instructions).

- Do some exercise (see chapter 15) or consider some vital energy
  exercises such as yoga, t'ai chi or psychocalisthenics (see Resources
  section). Exercise improves the circulation and oxygenates the
  blood, which is a natural high in itself, increasing your energy level
  and also helping you to relax properly.

- Put on some stimulating music and boogie to the beat (but not too
  loud, you don't want to scare your baby!).

- Maximise the light in your room with natural or full-spectrum light-
  ing, or take a walk outside in the daylight.

- Swathe yourself in vibrant colours – even if it's just a scarf. Magenta,
  orange, red and white can all stimulate your mood.

- Scent your room with lemon, eucalyptus, cinnamon or peppermint.

You can buy aroma lamps, which warm essential oils in water over a candle, evaporating their scent into the air.

● Have sex! This is an instant energiser. As long as it's not uncomfortable for you (and you may need to experiment with different positions to find the best way as you become more pregnant), you won't harm the baby.

Increase relaxation and reduce stress

Relaxation is vital to your health, especially now you're pregnant and there's someone else to consider. When we experience stress, we set in motion a chain of physical events that release hormones such as adrenalin to equip us to deal with a potentially dangerous situation. However, unlike our prehistoric ancestors, the stressful situations of today don't involve squaring up to a snarling beast or running away from a predator. We don't need to 'fight or flee' while we're stuck in traffic or having to deal with another automated customer service phone system (although we may feel like it!). But our bodies still react to stress in the same way. And while this is designed to ensure our survival, repeated stress reactions can impact negatively on our health.

In the short term, stress suppresses the immune system, slows down the body's rate of repair and metabolism and depletes stores of vital nutrients – all of which affect your developing baby. Research has found that high levels of stress and anxiety during pregnancy are associated with lower birth-weight and premature delivery. According to an American study, pregnant women experiencing high stress during pregnancy were four times more likely to deliver their babies prematurely than women who experienced little stress.[19] In another study, the risk of very low birth-weight is one-and-a-half times greater if the mother perceived that she 'almost always' felt stressed during her pregnancy.[20]

Long term, stress also promotes rapid ageing and weight gain, and can lead to chronic fatigue. So, learning to let go of stress and relax is crucial to both your own health and that of your developing baby. But now that having a drink or a cigarette as a way to wind down after a difficult day are off the agenda, how can you relax?

Take a deep breath

When you are stressed out, one of the quickest ways to regain balance is to breathe deeply and gain some perspective on whatever is making you feel anxious. Breathing deeply also brings more oxygen into your body, and consequently more energy. By regularly doing the following conscious breathing exercise, you can let go of stress, rebalance your mind and revitalise your body.

1. Sit comfortably, in a quiet place with your spine straight.

2. Focus your attention on your toes to check they are relaxed and take a deep breath in then out again to release any tension. Repeat this going up your body to your calves, thighs, buttocks, stomach, etc. until you reach your shoulders, neck, jawline and forehead.

3. When your body is fully relaxed, start to focus on breathing deeply. Take a deep breath into the base of your belly, letting it expand fully as you inhale slowly and deeply. Feel your diaphragm being pulled down towards the belly as your lungs fill with air from the bottom to the top. When you exhale, relax both your belly and your diaphragm, emptying your lungs from top to bottom.

4. When you have established a rhythm, start to count your out breaths from one to ten. When you reach ten, start again at one and repeat three times (i.e. for thirty breaths in total). If you lose count, just start that set again.

This exercise is best done each day for about five to ten minutes and again if you become stressed or upset during the day (but then only for one set of ten breaths).

Instant stress busters

There are entire sections in bookshops and libraries dedicated to books about stress management – indeed Patrick has written one himself (*Natural High Chill*, see Resources). So if you find that stress is a constant problem, you may want to investigate these self-help options further. In the meantime, here are some easy ways to destress and relax:

- Have a massage – a great way to release tension and bring about a feeling of wellbeing. Many therapists offer special pregnancy massages – ask at your local ante-natal classes or contact your local National Childbirth Trust (see the Resources section for details).

- Learn to meditate – often considered the reserve of monks and 'space cadets', meditation is actually a practical tool you can use to manage the stresses of daily living and stay relaxed. It works by expanding your awareness beyond the mind and body, promoting a feeling of calm and contentment. There are countless meditation approaches and courses available (check out local alternative health centres or do an internet search for courses in your area).

- Listen to some relaxing tunes – music has an immediate effect on how you feel. Musicians the world over have discovered certain beats, tones and melodies that can instantly relax and destress you. Obviously, what you like depends on your own personal taste, but if you need some inspiration, try Salve Regina's *Gregorian Chant*, Strauss's *Blue Danube*, Albinoni's *Adagios*, Vivaldi's *Four Seasons* or Various Artists' *Café Del Mar*.

- Tune into nature – whether it's a walk in the hills, the woods, along the water's edge or even in the park, nature has an extraordinary ability to bring you back to centre and relax you.

CHAPTER FIFTEEN

Getting Fit Not Fat

THE LAST THING you want to do in pregnancy is put your feet up and start eating more. Doing some regular exercise and keeping fit will give you much more energy and will also equip you better for giving birth, as well as being of benefit to your baby's health.

Without exercise, the body loses muscle tone and accumulates tension – and you feel tired. Exercise improves the circulation and oxygenates the blood, increasing your energy levels and also helping you to relax properly. That is why you sleep much better after swimming or a good, long walk.

If you were already doing exercise on a regular basis, there is no reason to stop now you're pregnant. Whether it's running, swimming, aerobics or dance classes, keep it up. These are all excellent 'aerobic' exercises if done properly, which means they cause your body to take in and use oxygen more efficiently. This improves the health of your heart and arteries, which is all good news for your baby. Giving birth has been likened, in terms of sheer physical exertion, to running a marathon. And, of course, the longer the labour the harder you work. So it pays to be aerobically fit.

Exercise for your baby's health too

Even if you haven't done much exercise before becoming pregnant, researchers have found that by starting, you can increase your chances of giving birth to a healthy baby. A study compared women doing moderate weight-bearing exercise, such as jogging or brisk walking, three to five times a week from their eighth week of pregnancy with those doing none at all. Babies born to the women who exercised were significantly heavier and longer than those whose mothers did no exercise (see page 138). In addition, the placenta grew faster and functioned better in those who exercised.[21]

Exercise may even seem easier during pregnancy. According to Dr James Clapp, who led the exercise research study, pregnancy induces a 'marked training effect' where the heart pumps more blood and the lungs take in more air. Contrary to what some believe, he says that exercise does not induce early labour, and it reduces distress in your baby.

Of course, if you have a complication with your pregnancy, you should talk to your doctor or midwife before rushing to the gym. But if your pregnancy is problem free, the ideal exercise programme would be doing a weight-bearing activity, such as jogging or aerobic dancing, for thirty continuous minutes three or four times a week.

If you are generally unfit, start with some gentle exercise and build up slowly. Perhaps go for a brisk walk several times a week, preferably involving the odd hill. Then start swimming or attending beginner aerobics classes, leaving out the hard bits. Remember too that exercise should be fun, so choose something you enjoy.

A note of caution

While keeping fit is important, avoid any exercise that could cause you physical trauma such as bumps or falls, as this could increase your risk of miscarriage. Going skiing for the first time or taking up abseiling or hand gliding are therefore unwise! The risk of injury to joints is also

greater in pregnancy, for two reasons. The extra weight you are carrying puts more of a strain on the weight-bearing joints (your hips,
knees and ankles) as well as your back. Also, the hormonal changes in
pregnancy loosen ligaments as this helps to free up the pelvis (vital for
delivering the baby), so you could more easily dislocate a joint during
pregnancy. But if you exercise sensibly and listen to your body, you
shouldn't experience any problems.

You can go on exercising in pregnancy until your body tells you to
stop. The fitter you are, the later this will be. In fact many people exercise right up to the end of pregnancy. Usually it is not the physical
inability that stops people exercising, but feeling tired.

Keeping active generally will also help you to stay fit. So take the
stairs when you can, get up to change the TV channel rather than
using the remote control, walk to the shops instead of taking the car
or bus and do all those little jobs you want to do around the house or
garden that you won't be able to do with a young baby around. On the
Better Pregnancy Diet and Supplement Plan, you'll have plenty of
energy to use up so make the most of it!

Strengthen your stomach and pelvic floor muscles

During pregnancy the abdominal muscles get severely stretched and
unless you do some form of exercise to maintain abdominal muscle
tone, you are more likely to suffer from backache, have a harder time
in labour, and end up with a bigger belly after the event.

If your current exercise programme doesn't include abdominal
exercises it is worth setting aside five minutes of every day to
strengthen these muscles. Ideally, you should learn any new exercise
from a professional instructor, so visit a gym or attend a yoga or exercise class. There are also lots of classes that are run especially for pregnant women, so check out your local paper for details. However, it's
not recommended to exercise in a horizontal position after the first
three months of pregnancy because this directs blood flow away from
the baby.

It's also a good idea to incorporate a pelvic floor exercise into your daily routine. This will help to strengthen the muscles of the birth canal, giving you more strength when you have to push. To discover where your pelvic floor muscles are, stop the flow of urine when you are passing water – you will feel the muscles contracting then relaxing as you let the urine flow again. If you stop and start the flow continually, you will be exercising your pelvic floor. This action of continually clenching and releasing your pelvic floor can be done completely discreetly while sitting at a desk or even waiting for a bus. It's also a good exercise to do after your baby is born to tone up your vagina.

PART THREE

YOUR GUIDE TO BEING A SUPER MUM

Now the wait is over and you finally have your baby in your arms. Although you've had nine months to get used to the idea, this can often be an overwhelming time. In this part of the book, we show you how to get off to a great start to motherhood, both for yourself and your baby, including:

- How to bounce back from the birth.
- Why breast feeding is the best option.
- How to ensure your milk optimally nourishes your baby.
- Which formulas are best if you cannot breast feed.
- How to deal with common problems that can occur in both you and your baby.
- What to do about vaccinations.

CHAPTER SIXTEEN

After Birth Revitalisers

G IVING BIRTH IS extremely hard work and the chances are you will be very tired afterwards, even if you are experiencing an after birth 'high'. So do accept any help that's offered from new grannies, uncles, aunts and friends, as you will need to conserve all your energy for the forthcoming weeks of disturbed nights.

If you have to stay in hospital for more than a day or so, it's unlikely the food you'll be offered will be the best for aiding recovery or boosting your energy, so ask family and friends to bring you in some healthy snacks. Fresh fruit, almonds, pumpkin and sunflower seeds, some oatcakes with nut butter, a cool bag with a vitality-packed salad or some hummus and carrot/celery sticks, for example, will all provide vital nutrients.

When you do go home, don't be tempted to rush around tidying up or cooking. You need to conserve your energy for recovering and looking after your new baby. Arrange for your partner to stock the fridge and when friends or relatives come, don't be afraid to ask them to help too. People love to feel useful, so they'll be happy to do some shopping, cook a meal or make a big batch of homemade soup (a mixed vegetable soup with lentils or organic chicken can be a meal in itself). You could also ask someone to scrub a big bag of baking potatoes, so you can just pop one in the oven to eat whenever you fancy (see page 116 for easy fillings and other quick meal ideas).

If you are breast feeding, you need to eat an extra 500 calories a day (that's 25 per cent more than before you got pregnant), so make sure you eat regularly and eat well – now your baby is born, your diet still needs to nourish both of you. Also, drink plenty of fluid and get lots of rest – if you become dehydrated, over- tired or stressed, your milk supply can be affected. As you'll be having broken nights, try to nap during the day to catch up on lost sleep.

If your partner has to go back to work straight away, it's a good idea to arrange for someone to spend the first week or so with you, so you're not worrying alone about how often you should change your baby's nappy or whether demand feeding really means every thirty minutes!

Help yourself to heal

Giving birth is hugely physically demanding. If you've had a vaginal birth, you are probably feeling sore, especially if you've torn or had stitches. And if you've had a Caesarean, remember you're recovering from major surgery and it will be six to eight weeks before you can return to normal activities such as lifting or driving. Getting the right nutrients will help you speed up the healing process. So continue with the healthy diet you've been eating while pregnant and take the supplements outlined later (page 156) for the first two weeks. Vitamins A, C, E and zinc are particularly key to repairing damaged tissues (you can also use vitamin E topically on stretch marks or scars – see opposite), as are essential fats, so make sure you eat foods rich in these nutrients – fresh vegetables and fruit, fish, nuts and seeds are all good sources (see chapter 10 for detailed listings). These will also provide plenty of fibre – if you're sore down below, you certainly don't want the discomfort of constipation to deal with too! The amino acid glutamine is particularly effective for mending cuts and wounds, especially after surgery – take 5g three times a days twenty minutes before eating (i.e. on an empty stomach) until you've healed (see the Resources section for supplier details). The homoeopathic remedy arnica is also useful for bruising – it's quite safe to take while breast feeding and can even be beneficial to your baby, as its healing properties will be carried in your milk to help him or her recover from the birth too. You can buy this from good chemists and healthfood shops.

Special nutrient needs

Because giving birth is so physically demanding, it's also nutritionally demanding and your stores of vitamins and minerals will have been fully called upon. Leading up to the birth, you will transfer vital nutrients to your baby to prepare them for life outside your womb. The essential fat DHA, for example, is needed in large amounts for your baby's continued brain development, as is zinc. So if you haven't been getting a good supply yourself, you're likely to become deficient and this can lead to post-natal depression (see page 169 for more on this). The physical act of giving birth will also drain you of key vitamins and minerals – zinc again is lost during any demanding event, plus iron with blood loss, B vitamins are lost with all that energy you've expended, and calcium and magnesium are depleted by hours of muscle contractions. Our ancestors and most other mammals found the perfect ready-made solution to replenish all these lost nutrients – eating the placenta! However, while this is still practised in some parts of the world, it is no longer commonplace in Western society. So, if placenta stew doesn't appeal, luckily we have multivitamin and mineral supplements that are far easier to swallow!

We've already mentioned zinc, iron, calcium, magnesium and B vitamins. Vitamin C will also be depleted, and A and E are key. As already outlined, vitamin A is vital for any bruising and wound healing and will help restore your abdomen, uterus and vagina to their former size. Vitamin E helps healing too, but most of all, together with vitamin C, it encourages skin elasticity and the contraction of skin across the abdomen. Applying vitamin E oil directly to a stretch mark or scar (if you've had a Caesarean) will also help to heal the skin – just burst open a capsule and rub the contents into the skin. Alternatively you can use a strong vitamin E cream.

Your revitalising supplement plan

Up until the birth, you've probably already been taking the supplement plan we recommended in chapter 12. So, to keep it simple, we've just increased the dosage and added in an antioxidant, if you haven't already been taking one, to boost levels of all the nutrients you need to bounce back to superhealth (see below). Follow this programme for two weeks, then revert back to your pregnancy level to sustain you through breast feeding. Obviously during this time you'll have a lot on your plate, so we suggest you prepare your 'two-week supplement plan' in advance and put each day's supply into fourteen small bags or envelopes that you can easily pack into your hospital bag and leave by the kettle to take when you get home.

Supplement	Breakfast	Lunch	Dinner
Multivitamin and mineral	1	1	1
Vitamin C (1,000mg)	1	1	1
Antioxidant	1	1	1
Essential fats			
(400mg EPA/			
200mg DHA/			
200mg GLA)	1	1	1
Optional:			
Glutamine	5g	5g	5g

See the Resources section at the back for supplier details.

Vitamin K protects your baby

Vitamin K is vital for blood clotting and if there's a deficiency, bleeding can occur. In a newborn baby, this is called haemorrhagic disease and it affects about 1 in 10,000 babies. As a result, it's become standard medical practice to give all newborn babies a vitamin K injection. However, some research has linked this with an increased risk of childhood cancers,[1] so now it's more commonly offered by mouth. The exact quantity a newborn needs isn't really understood with different doses given by different hospitals, and it's not really known whether this is harmful or not. Our advice therefore is to ensure your diet is rich in vitamin K food sources such as cauliflower, broccoli and cabbage so that when you breast feed, you will naturally pass on vitamin K in your milk. This way there is no need for your baby to have an injection or oral supplement – unless he or she is identified as being particularly at risk at birth. So put coleslaw, cauliflower cheese and broccoli soup on your menu for the first few weeks after giving birth. After this time, levels should have risen and the healthy bacteria that colonise your baby's gut (which is sterile at birth) will start to produce sufficient levels of their own. Incidentally, vitamin K is added to formula milk, so even if you don't breast feed, you baby will still be getting a good supply.

In summary:

- **Regain** your energy with energy-giving foods and not stodgy nutrient-depleted foods that will make you more tired.

- **Don't** be afraid to accept help and support – you will be tired and need to rest.

- **Speed** up the healing process and take extra supplements to replenish what's been lost in childbirth and help to mend sore tissues.

- **Exercise** your right to choose whether the baby receives vitamin K supplementation – and boost your levels through diet if you want to breast feed.

CHAPTER SEVENTEEN

Breast is Definitely Best

EIGHTY YEARS AGO this chapter would not have been needed, as breast feeding was the norm. However, the number of women who choose to breast feed has declined so much that now women have to be persuaded back into it. Some don't want the inconvenience and some want to get back to work quickly. Some experience pain when the milk comes in the first week. This goes away if you persist. But, as you will see, there is high price to pay for this short-term gain.

Others fear that they won't be able to do it – that their breasts are too small or that they won't produce enough milk, but breast size has little to do with your ability to feed and, as long as you're well nourished, your milk supply will meet your baby's needs. As with learning any new skill, it can be difficult and sometimes painful at first, but it's worth persisting as there are so many advantages to breast feeding and, every week, the media seem to report another long-term benefit.

The benefits for your baby

- Breast-fed babies are healthier. Breast milk contains antibodies that are not found in formula milk and these offer your baby protection against infections. The first type of milk you produce – colostrum –

is particularly rich in antibodies, protein and nutrients, which offer enhanced protection and nourishment for the first few days of your baby's life. A study by doctors at the University of California, the University of Rochester and the American Pediatrics' Center for Child Health Research found that 'babies breast fed for at least six months after birth are much less likely to develop pneumonia, colds and ear infections'. Other research has found that breast-fed babies suffer with fewer gastric complaints and are less prone to allergies in later life.[2]

- Breast-fed babies are brainier. A recent series of studies conducted world-wide indicate they have an IQ of 6–10 points higher than formula-fed babies.[3] This is probably due to the high levels of the essential fat DHA found in breast milk, which is vital for brain development.

- The fat-soluble vitamins in breast milk are more easily absorbed. In a Brazilian study, only 1 in 176 breast-fed babies had lower than adequate levels of vitamin E, compared to more than half in a cow's milk formula-fed group.[4] Another study has shown that breast milk is higher in vitamin D than formula milk – and not just any vitamin D, but a particular kind, which has been found to be two-and-a-half times more effective at preventing rickets (a deficiency disease where bones don't develop properly, which, amazingly, is on the increase in Britain).[5]

- There are more minerals in breast milk. Formula milks contain no selenium (a vital immune booster) or chromium (which helps to balance blood sugar, i.e. energy levels) and the manganese (needed for healthy bones) in breast milk is twenty times more absorbable than that in formulas.[6] Calcium, iron and zinc are also better absorbed from breast milk.

- Breast milk helps to establish healthy gut bacteria – a type of beneficial gut bacteria called bifido bacteria is present in breast but not formula milk and this protects against harmful bacteria invading your baby's digestive tract and also helps prevent colic and eczema developing.

- Breast-fed babies are less likely to be obese. A study of 32,000 Scottish children aged three to four found that those breast fed for six to eight weeks after birth were 30 per cent less likely to be obese than children who were bottle fed.[7]

- Sucking on a breast is much harder work than sucking on a bottle. So breast-fed babies develop a much stronger jaw, which stands them in good stead for when they start eating solids and developing speech.

The benefits for you

- Convenience and cost – no bottles to sterilise or formula milk to prepare, warm or pay for (it's estimated you save around £450 in the first year).[8]

- Breast feeding helps you lose any excess weight – because your baby is consuming about 500 calories a day, even when you're eating more, you're likely to find shifting any extra pounds is far easier.

- Suckling promotes the release of the hormone oxytocin, which stimulates your uterus to contract back it its pre-birth size.

- Breast feeding reduces your risk of developing breast cancer – the rate is 22 per cent lower among pre-menopausal women who breast fed for between four and twelve months, and the longer you feed and the more children you have the more the risk is reduced.[9]

And the disadvantages?

We've established a strong case for breast over bottle feeding. However, there are a few downsides. Because breast milk is far more easily digestible, your baby will need feeding more often than a formula-fed baby, and this can be especially hard at night during the first few months. You are also on call all the time and can't delegate feeding to anyone else (unless of course you express milk which can be put in a bottle – handy when you need the night off). Your milk is only as good as your nutrient intake, so your diet and supplement programme needs to be optimum (see later). And you must continue to avoid the foods and drinks that were off limits while you were pregnant, which are outlined in chapter 11 (although you can enjoy the occasional glass of wine). But these are minor inconveniences compared to the many benefits of breast feeding. And the time span is relatively short – after nine months of pregnancy, what's another six to give your baby the very best start in life?

How often should you feed your baby?

If you let your baby feed whenever he or she wants to (including at night), you are far more likely to get a good supply of milk going without suffering breast engorgement or sore nipples. Some research suggests that fewer than five feeds a day will not keep an adequate milk supply going, so if you feel like you are constantly feeding your baby, you are probably doing the right thing! Unlike bottle feeding, breast feeding is hard to regulate – the amount your baby suckles cannot be carefully measured, so there's little point trying to regiment how long he or she spends at each breast. Different babies also suck at different rates – some are slower and others guzzle. It's also impossible to over-feed a breast-fed baby. So don't be concerned – after you've got the hang of it, you'll know what feels right. But if you need help to get started or do run into problems, contact your local breast-feeding group, for instance the National Childbirth Trust or La Leche League (see the Resources section for contact details).

Looking after your own needs

Looking after yourself is key, as the quality of your breast milk depends on your diet and wellbeing. This means getting adequate nutrients, eating enough to get the 500 extra calories your baby will consume, and getting enough rest.

It is important to ensure an adequate protein intake, particularly if you are not eating meat. If you feel you're not producing enough milk or your baby seems to be constantly suckling without being satisfied, eating more protein should help. One study showed that increasing the amount of protein in the diet increased the milk supply and consequently the size of the babies.[10]

However, there's no need to gorge on steaks and cheese. Follow the advice for the Better Pregnancy Diet – but eat more often. That may mean three meals a day plus two or three snacks. Even if you've gained weight during pregnancy, breast feeding will quickly burn up your fat reserves, so as long as you're eating healthily and not filling up on empty calories such as cakes, sweets or biscuits (which contribute calories but not enough nutrients, so won't in fact benefit you or your baby), you'll have enough energy and lose weight. The same advice applies to foods to avoid (chapter 11), as you can still pass on food poisoning bacteria through your milk. And try to eat organic as any pesticides and chemicals will be passed to your baby via your breast milk.

Getting enough liquid is just as important as getting enough food. Your baby will be taking between ½ to 1 litre (1 to 2 pints) of water through your breast milk, which needs to be replaced. This means drinking around 3 litres (just over 5 pints) a day. As most substances cross into your breast milk in varying degrees of concentration, it is important not to drink coffee, chocolate, cola drinks or any other drink containing sugar or artificial additives. You also don't need to drink milk to make milk, so don't be concerned if it doesn't suit you. Choose healthy alternatives such as herb teas, coffee substitutes (available from healthfood shops), fruit juice diluted half and half with water, sparkling mineral water or filtered/bottled water. If you are drinking enough you should not have to give your baby extra water, unless advised to do so by a doctor if your baby is constipated, has a fever or diarrhoea, or is vomiting. Breast milk really is a complete food for your baby.

You can start to drink alcohol again in moderation – but no more than a few glasses of wine a week. It's best to have it after you've given your baby his or her last main feed of the day so by the time you give the night feed, the alcohol will have begun to dissipate. However, if your baby gets colic, hiccups or appears to react, you should stop having any alcohol at all.

Does breast feeding guarantee good nutrition?

A mother's milk is only as good as the mother. And as we've seen in chapter 12, eating the best diet still doesn't provide all the nutrients we need. Even the government accepts that babies need extra nutrients – which is why baby vitamin drops are available free from your doctor. However, these are unnecessary if you supplement your own diet so your milk's nutrient content is enhanced.

So, after you've finished the supplement programme recommended for the first two weeks (page 156), we suggest you revert to the supplement plan for pregnancy outlined in chapter 12. This will continue to provide optimal levels of the vitamins, minerals and essential fats you need in sufficient quantity to make sure your milk meets your baby's needs. The levels are deliberately higher than the RDA (see page 98) – as studies show even mothers consuming close to the RDA don't necessarily produce milk that then provides the recommended levels of nutrients for their baby.

For example, in a study women consuming an average of 1.8mg of B6 (just below the RDA of 2mg) were supplemented with 20mg of B6 (twenty times the RDA) and still only produced a maximum of 0.28mg of the 0.3mg needed by their babies. In other words, even this level of supplementation didn't meet their baby's basic needs for B6.[11] This is why supplements of 50mg of B6 are recommended while breast feeding to reach optimal levels. However, doses in excess of 200mg a day have been reported to suppress milk production, so don't take more than 50mg.

While too much of a certain nutrient may affect you, there appears to be a mechanism to stop the baby getting more than they need. A study of mothers supplementing 1,000mg of vitamin C, for example, showed that their milk provided between 40mg and 86mg a day – and this didn't increase when higher levels were supplemented.[12]

One nutrient that is nearly always deficient in breast milk is zinc. A newborn infant up to six months needs 3mg of zinc a day. Yet the average amount supplied daily in human milk is only 1.3mg during the first three months and even less, only 0.6mg a day, in the second three months of breast feeding. So mothers and babies alike become increasingly deficient as breast feeding continues. However, breast-milk zinc is generally far better absorbed than dietary zinc, so these low figures may not necessarily equate to serious zinc deficiency. Nevertheless, you need to get 25mg of zinc a day while breast feeding, and that means supplementing 15mg.

If you are vegan, you need to ensure you get enough vitamin D. As vitamin D is only found in animal foods, you may wish to consider taking a cod liver oil supplement just for the duration that you breast feed, or giving a quarter of a teaspoon to your baby (you can even rub it into his or her skin). Alternatively, make sure you get exposure to natural light three times a week, as this synthesises vitamin D in your skin. B12 is another vitamin that's often lacking in a vegan diet. To boost levels, eat fortified cereals, yeast extract, non-dairy milks or fermented soya products.

How long to breast feed for

Research suggests that the longer you breast feed, the better it is for both your and your baby's health. But as we've seen, being optimally nourished is key to the quality of your milk. Our advice is follow the diet and supplement plan in this book and breast feed exclusively for four to six months, then reduce as you start to introduce your baby to solid foods, continuing with supplementary feeds until your baby is about a year old. While 'mixed' feeding may be tempting – for example making your baby's last feed of the day a bottle feed so they sleep for longer – research shows that this can increase your baby's risk of developing allergies and impair his or her mental and nervous development. However, if you have to go back to work, try to continue giving breast feeds morning and night. Again, your local breast-feeding group will be able to show you how to manage your milk flow to enable you to do this without too much discomfort, and can also advise on expressing milk effectively.

What if I can't breast feed?

Not all women have the choice of whether or not to breast feed their babies. So if you can't, which formula is best?

Although we have advanced from the days when cow's milk was boiled, diluted and had sugar added to it, we have still not produced a formula milk that is identical to human milk. In fact, the initial reasons for giving babies cow's milk half a century ago are unclear, as donkey's milk actually resembles human milk far more closely. Cows were, however, much more available and produce more milk.

Today, you can buy cow, goat and soya formulas and each is modified to suit a baby's immature digestion. While cow's milk is still the most widely used, some babies are allergic to it. Goat's milk is a less allergenic alternative because it's more easily digested. Although similar in nutritional content to cow's milk, the leading UK make, Nanny, is fortified with extra vitamins and minerals and has a superior essential fat content to cow's milk. However, if you are not using Nanny, you will need to check that your source is boiled or pasteurised and from herds tested for brucellosis and tuberculosis.

The second alternative to cow's milk is soya milk, but this is only recommended for babies allergic to both cow and goat's milk (although soya itself is a common allergen). Because soya is dairy free, it doesn't contain lactose (a milk sugar) so glucose syrup is often the main ingredient and this can damage developing teeth. Soya formulas also contain natural hormone-like substances called phytoestrogens and there is some concern that these may affect a baby's hormone balance, although others believe they actually have a protective effect. The last concern links soya milk with an increased risk of developing a peanut allergy. Researchers at the University of Bristol monitored 14,000 babies from birth and found that almost a quarter of those who went on to develop this allergy had been given soya formula in their first two years. However, to put this in perspective, of these 14,000, only 49 developed the allergy. So if your child has to have soya, just be cautious when weaning (see chapter 20) and be careful when introducing peanuts. By the way, there's no evidence that, if you eat soya foods, this predisposes your baby to allergy.

Selecting the right formula

Once you've decided which type of milk to feed your baby, you then need to choose a brand. Prepare to be bamboozled as there are a great many to choose from! However, rather than list the many different makes, it's better to know what to look for.

- First you'll want to avoid formulas that contain added sugar, glucose or corn syrup. They simply aren't needed. Lactose (milk sugar) is what sweetens breast milk, and should ideally be used in formula milk too (although lactose isn't used in soya formulas).

- Organic milks are preferable to non-organic. Babynat, for example, is a good organic formula available in the UK and much of Europe. Nanny goat formula is made from free-range goats.

- Consider nutrient content. All formula milk is required by law to add essential vitamins and minerals, but the quantity can vary. Probably the easiest way to pick out a good formula milk is to compare the zinc content. The higher the better. It should also contain manganese, chromium and selenium, although many don't. The amino acid taurine is also now added to some formulas as it's believed to help replicate the sleepiness babies experience after breast milk and may also be essential for babies. New guidelines state that infant formulas must contain some essential fats, but look at what and how much is included. DHA and AA are both vital for brain and nervous system development.

There are a number of myths about formula milks. The manufacturers will try to tell you that you need to change formulas once a baby is three months old. This is totally unnecessary. It is far better to choose a good formula, get your baby used to it and stick with it. Some mothers are tempted to make a more concentrated solution than instructed because they think the milk looks too thin. This is extremely dangerous, as you can overload your baby's kidneys, which can cause fits or even death. So follow the instructions exactly.

Boosting a formula-fed baby's nutrition

In the same way as we suggest you supplement your diet if you breast feed, we recommend you supplement your baby's diet if you bottle feed. This way you can compensate for some of the inadequacies of formula milks and help to give your baby a better start in life.

- Establishing healthy gut bacteria is important to reduce the risk of digestive upsets, colic, eczema and even asthma but the bacteria of breast milk is lacking in formula milk. So add a quarter of a teaspoon of an infant probiotic (again, see the Resources section for supplier details) once a day to your warmed bottle of formula (don't add before heating as the process will kill the beneficial bacteria).

- If your formula doesn't have any selenium or chromium, add a few drops of liquid mineral formula to a bottle once a day. Likewise, if vitamin levels are low, you can add a few liquid vitamin drops too. The quantity will vary according to the brand you use, but see Resources section for details.

In summary, to ensure your breast milk is optimal:

- **You** should continue with the Better Pregnancy Diet but eat more often. So have three main meals plus three snacks in between. Be sure to get enough protein, and try to continue eating organic wherever possible.

- **Drink** plenty of fluid – aim for 3 litres (just over 5 pints) a day as water, herb teas, diluted juices. Avoid caffeinated drinks, such as coffee and colas, and limit your consumption of tea to no more than three cups a day and alcohol to just a few glasses of wine a week.

- **Continue** to supplement your diet – with the plan outlined on page 156 for the first two weeks, then revert back to your pregnancy supplement programme for the remaining time you are breast feeding.

- **Get** plenty of rest.

If you are bottle feeding:

- **Do** your homework before choosing a formula.

- **Supplement** your baby with extra essential fats, probiotics and minerals.

~

CHAPTER EIGHTEEN

Preventing Problems in Mother and Baby: from Sore Nipples to Nappy Rash

Y OUR BODY UNDERGOES huge upheaval during pregnancy and birth, so it's perfectly normal for you to experience a few problems settling into motherhood. Your baby has been through a lot too – being built from scratch in just nine months, then going through labour with you and having to adjust to the outside world, so he or she will be sensitive to their new environment. However, with the right nutrition, you can usually put any problems right to ensure you're both in the peak of health.

Troubleshooters for you

Avoid the baby blues

Serious post-natal depression is thought to affect up to 15 per cent of new mothers, and feeling weepy or down is even more common. Although there's a psychological component – now you have the huge responsibility of a baby – post-natal depression is usually triggered by hormonal and chemical changes that can be supported with good nutrition.

Before you give birth, you transfer a large supply of zinc to your baby, and if you didn't have a good supply yourself, the chances are you're now deficient, especially if your labour was long and difficult or you had a Caesarean. Depression is a common side effect of zinc deficiency, as are white marks on more than two finger-nails, a poor appetite, stretch marks and a poor immune system. So if you have any of these additional symptoms, up your supplementary zinc intake to 15mg twice a day until your mood improves. As zinc works with the B vitamin family, particularly B6, also take a B complex supplement (see the Resources section for suppliers). Dr Carl Pfeiffer, the world's leading authority on treating mental health problems with nutrition, says 'We have never seen post-natal depression or psychosis in any of our patients treated with zinc and B6'.

The other common deficiency in post-natal depression is essential fats. In a study of 11,721 British women, those who consumed fish two or three times a week were half as likely to suffer from depression as women with the lowest intakes.[13] So eat more oily fish (but see page 31 for cautions) and make sure you continue eating seeds daily (see page 84), as well as taking the essential fat supplement outlined on page 84.

Banish breast discomfort

When you start breast feeding, it's common for your nipples to get sore. You can help to prevent this by ensuring your baby is latching on properly (which you can be taught at local breast-feeding classes – see the Resources section). Your nipples will soon toughen up, but if your breasts become really sore, don't grin and bear it – do something, as if left, your milk ducts can become infected and mastitis can develop. Putting a green cabbage leaf inside your bra may sound like an old wives' tale, but cabbage is rich in healing glutamine and can really bring relief, especially if you chill it first then bash it to release its healing enzymes. Applying vitamin E oil will soothe cracked nipples – just prick a capsule and gently rub the contents in. And if your breasts become engorged, either feed your baby (even if you have to wake him or her up first) or express some milk to release the pressure. Also make sure you are getting plenty of rest between feeds and following the revitalising supplement plan (page 56) for the first few weeks of breast feeding.

TLC for stretch marks

Vitamins A, C, E and the mineral zinc are all key for skin health. A stretch mark is a tear in the collagen fibre of your skin, so while these nutrients can't necessarily repair it, they can help increase skin elasticity and tone, and prevent any further stretch marks developing. Applying vitamin E oil directly to the stretch mark or scar (if you've had a Caesarean) will help to reduce the visible marks – just prick a supplement capsule and rub the contents directly into the skin. Alternatively you can use a strong vitamin E cream.

Troubleshooters for your baby

Ease colic

Babies with colic experience similar symptoms to adults with irritable bowel syndrome (IBS) – muscle spasms and pain, often occurring in the evening, with continuous crying only alleviated (sometimes after hours of discomfort) by passing wind or a bowel movement. Colic is most common during the first few months and it usually passes by the time a baby reaches four months. What you're feeding your baby is usually the cause. If breast feeding, then check your diet to see if you can identify any common triggers – dairy, chocolate, coffee, spicy foods, nightshades (tomatoes, peppers, aubergine, potatoes), citrus fruits and cucumbers can all be culprits. Gas-forming foods, such as onions, beans, cauliflower, broccoli and Brussels sprouts, can also make colic worse, so turn detective and eliminate or rotate possible irritants. Seek the support of a nutritional therapist if you need help with this.

If bottle feeding, a cow's milk allergy may be the cause, so either switch to a whey-based formula (whey is easier to digest then casein, which is added to some formulas) or try your baby on goat's milk formula (see page 165). Alternatively, you could try adding lactase drops (available from good healthfood shops) to your baby's bottle a few hours before feeding – this enzyme will start to pre-digest the lactose in the milk and help to ease irritation. Adding an infant-formulated probiotic can also help ease digestive discomfort (see the guidelines given for eczema below), as can chamomile, fennel, ginger or peppermint tea. If breast feeding, drink a cup twice a day (experiment with each or a combination to see which suits your baby best) or add a teaspoon of diluted tea three times a day to your baby's bottle until the colic eases. If you have no joy, try increasing the dose – Israeli researchers found that the symptoms of colic reduced in more than half of a group of babies who were given half a cup of a mixed tea (chamomile, liquorice, fennel and mint) each day.[14] Finally, check feeding position to ensure your baby isn't swallowing too much air, and gently massage your baby's tummy and move his or her legs in a pedalling motion to release trapped wind several times a day.

Eliminate eczema

Skin irritation in you or your baby is often a sign that you or they are (a) reacting negatively to something (i.e. a food or chemical such as washing powder), (b) are not getting enough essential nutrients (usually essential fats) or (c) have an imbalance in gut bacteria. So, first, if you're breast feeding check your diet and eliminate common allergens – wheat and dairy, then tea, coffee, chocolate, citrus, soya, nuts, eggs, gluten grains (wheat, oats, rye, barley) for a week. Then reintroduce them one at a time, with a new food every three days, and monitor the results. In this way you can usually pinpoint the offender. If you're bottle feeding, your baby could be reacting to the formula you're using. Follow the advice given on switching formula for colic (see previous section). Also switch to a non-allergenic washing powder and fabric softener. Next, or if this doesn't work, double your intake of essential fats (see page 84). This will be passed to your baby in your breast milk, but if you're bottle feeding, then add fish oil to the formula milk or rub it into your baby's skin (see page 167 for amounts). Finally, supplement your diet with probiotics (see Resources section) – take two capsules twenty minutes before eating three times a day – or add an infant probiotic to your baby's formula milk (see page 232). Research has found that giving pregnant or nursing mothers and their babies probiotics cuts the risk of childhood allergies such as eczema by 50 per cent.[15] If you still find no relief, contact a nutritional therapist who can examine the causes in more detail.

Minimise the risk of cot death

Every year, 300 babies in the UK die of cot death and the causes are not fully understood. Research throws up clues every so often – iron or lead toxicity and vitamin A deficiency have been linked, as has high maternal consumption of caffeine during pregnancy, and the risk is greater in households with a smoker, for example. Food allergy – especially to milk or gluten – is a possibility worth considering. Some also claim there's a link to vaccinations – either due to the toxic ingredients many vaccines contain, or their impact on a baby's immature immune system (see chapter 19 for more on this). But there doesn't appear to be any definitive answer. So what can you do? By following the Better Pregnancy Diet and supplement plan, you will be guarding against nutrient deficiencies in you, and will therefore minimise the risk of passing these on to your baby. Following the advice in chapter 3 will help to reduce both your and your baby's exposure to toxic substances (although we do recommend you having a hair mineral analysis to check your status before you conceive – see chapter 3 for details).

Most health experts now agree that the risk of cot death is reduced where a baby is put to sleep on his or her back and is not allowed to get too hot. The Foundation for the Study of Infant Deaths recommends parents use light blankets instead of bulky quilts and that a baby's head should not be covered while sleeping. The room where a baby sleeps should also be kept between 16 and 20°C.

We also recommend you use a BabySafe baby mattress protector (see the Resources section for details). This has been developed by a New Zealand chemist called Dr Jim Sprott who believes that the flame-retardant substances in baby mattresses give off toxic fumes when they come into contact with damp conditions (caused by a baby dribbling or vomiting, for example). His theory is that if these poisonous fumes don't disperse, they can build up until they reach a level where they can shut down the baby's central nervous system and heart function and breathing stops. But until you can buy a mattress cover (or when you can't use one, e.g. while travelling), elevate the head end of your baby's cot an inch or two so that any toxic gases can flow to the foot and dissipate.

Cure constipation

Constipation is rare in breast-fed babies, but if happens, check your diet for possible allergens (see the advice given for eczema) and make sure you are drinking 3 litres of fluid (just over 5 pints) a day. In bottle-fed babies, again suspect a reaction to the formula you are using, but before you switch, try increasing your baby's liquid intake, either by adding extra water to each feed or by giving a cooled, boiled water bottle. Probiotics may also help (see page 167). Persistent constipation should be investigated by a doctor or nutritional practitioner, as should any diarrhoea (which needs immediate medical attention).

Prevent nappy rash

Although common, nappy rash is not normal and can be avoided by eliminating any suspect foods that may be upsetting your baby (see page 172 for details). Ensure, too, that your breast milk is rich in the skin-healing nutrients vitamin A, C and E plus zinc and essential fats by boosting levels of these in your diet and supplement programme. And if you're bottle feeding, check for levels of these in your baby's formula and add them if necessary (see page 208). Cleanliness is obviously important, but also check that your baby is not reacting to anything in the wipes you are using. Try to leave off the nappy to air your baby's bottom each day and make sure it's really dry before putting another nappy back on.

❧

CHAPTER NINETEEN

What Your Doctor May Not Tell You About Vaccinations

VACCINATIONS ARE HERALDED as one of the wonders of our age, a triumph of modern medicine versus nature. Yet there are claims that they can damage rather than protect health, with examples of autism, disability, brain damage and even death given as side effects. Your child can receive up to twenty-five vaccinations by the age of fifteen months, with many given in their first six months of life. Obviously you don't want to expose your baby to unnecessary risks, so it's a good idea to take a closer look at the evidence.

A vaccination is based on the idea of introducing a dead or disabled infectious agent into a person, then allowing their immune system to respond and produce antibodies. The theory is that by 'memorising' the antigen and how to make the antibody, your immune system has an advantage in dealing with an infection, should you become exposed to the agent again, because it can act quickly.

The main issues regarding vaccinations are as follows:

1. How effective are they?

2. How dangerous is the disease?

3. How dangerous is the vaccine?

4. Are combination vaccines more dangerous?

5. When, if at all, is the best time to be vaccinated?

6. What are the alternatives to vaccination?

Vaccinations are less effective than you think

The scientific literature is far from conclusive on the success of vaccinations, with reports claiming anything from 20 to 90 per cent effectiveness, depending on the vaccine. The fact is many epidemic diseases come in cycles and have declined due to improvements in sanitation and isolation of those people infected with the disease.

A case in point is the 1870–2 Victorian smallpox epidemic in England. The outbreak claimed 44,000 lives, even though most of the population had been vaccinated. During the next outbreak in 1892, the town of Leicester decided against vaccination on the grounds that it didn't work, and instead relied only on sanitation and isolation. This outbreak saw just 19 cases and one death per 100,000. Nearby Warrington had six times as many cases and eleven times the death rate, even though 99 per cent of its population had been vaccinated.[16]

Similar inconsistencies in results with vaccinations are seen today. For example, in the US, the incidence of measles continued to rise all the way into the 1990s, despite the introduction of the vaccine in 1957. And in England in the 1970s, deaths from pertussis (whooping cough) dropped only after the vaccination rate reduced by 30 per cent.

Conversely, measles, mumps, smallpox, whooping cough, polio and meningitis outbreaks have all occurred in vaccinated populations. In 1989, the US Center for Disease Control (CDC) reported, 'Among school-aged children, [measles] outbreaks have occurred in schools with vaccination levels of greater than 98 per cent. [They] have occurred in all parts of the country, including areas that had not reported measles for years.' The CDC even reported a measles outbreak in a population that had been 100 per cent vaccinated. A study examining this outbreak concluded, 'The apparent paradox is that as measles immunisation rates rise to high levels in a population, measles becomes a disease of immunised persons.' However, there is no disputing the fact that since concerns over the MMR vaccination have caused immunisation levels to drop to below 75 per cent in some parts of the UK, outbreaks of measles have risen.

Finally, one of the apparent success stories for vaccination is polio. Yet, during a 1962 US Congressional hearing, Dr Bernard Greenberg, head of the Department of Biostatistics for the University of North Carolina School of Public Health, testified that the cases of polio not only increased after mandatory vaccinations – up 50 per cent from 1957 to 1958, and up 80 per cent from 1958 to 1959 – but that the statistics were deliberately manipulated by the Public Health Service to give the opposite impression.

Non-lethal diseases

Vaccinations are available for certain strains of microbes causing measles, mumps, chickenpox, rubella, diphtheria, whooping cough, tetanus, polio, meningitis, hepatitis and tuberculosis.

Arguably, some of these diseases are more life-threatening, and more prevalent, than others. For example, measles and mumps are very common, yet are rarely fatal, except in poorly nourished infants with compromised immune systems. Therefore, if your baby is optimally nourished, you can make a good case for delaying immunisation. If, by the time he or she reaches their teenage years and has still not contracted either disease (and so not conferred their own natural immunisation), you can then get them vaccinated, as measles and mumps can have more serious health implications in adults.

In the case of rubella, it makes sense to give the vaccine to girls early in their teenage years, as the disease can harm the unborn baby of a pregnant women. As for diphtheria, while it is more life-threatening, the chance of dying from the disease – with or without vaccination – is less than 1 in 100,000. In fact, many medical reports indicate that early vaccination confers little benefit.

Whooping cough and tetanus

According to Dr Gordon Stewart, one of Britain's top whooping cough experts, whooping cough is no longer a serious threat to the life and health of our children. There were no cases of brain damage or death among children during the last three outbreaks in the UK. However, the incidence of whooping cough in adults has gone up since the introduction of early immunisation, which may suggest that the vaccine is suppressing the disease.

Tetanus is even rarer. However, the risk is minimal and, when treated correctly, 80 per cent of people recover. Fortunately, tetanus can be easily controlled. The risk with this disease involves cutting yourself, then picking up the virus in manure or dirt – so while it's unlikely your baby will do this until he or she becomes mobile, young children may be more at risk when they start exploring. However, you can massively reduce this risk by cleaning wounds properly, and not allowing a wound to close until healing has occurred below the skin's surface. If you do decide to give your child a tetanus shot, keep in mind that the presence of the tetanus antibodies reduces rapidly after a vaccination. Therefore, you'll need to keep repeating it every five or so years to confer a degree of protection.

Polio

Polio is one vaccine that many authorities consider essential, yet contrary to public perception, vaccinations are less effective than you might think. Because vaccinations are for specific strains of polio microbes that are permanently evolving and changing, there's no guarantee of protection. For example, an outbreak of polio occurred in Taiwan, where 98 per cent of young children had been immunised.[17] In 1961, a polio outbreak in Massachusetts resulted in more cases of paralysis among those vaccinated than those who were not.[18] And another study found that three out of five Americans who had contracted polio during foreign travel had previously been vaccinated.[19]

And still, most authorities will highly recommend that your baby has a polio vaccine if you are taking him or her abroad. Our recommendation is that you first find out how common polio is in the country you are visiting. But if you are not planning to go abroad, it's really not necessary. For example, in the UK, there are no more than two cases per year. In fact, you are more likely to be hit by a double-decker bus than contracting polio in Britain!

Meningitis

One of the diseases that we do recommend vaccinating against is the *Haemophilus influenza* type B (Hib) virus, the most common cause of meningitis, which causes upper respiratory and ear infections, pneumonia and inflammation of the spinal cord. It most often affects babies between the ages of six to twelve months, with 75 per cent of all cases occurring before the age of two. Because a lack of hygiene in day care centres is partly blamed for the spread of the disease, if your baby is going to be looked after with other children, we definitely recommend vaccinating him or her with the Hib meningitis vaccine.

More recently the spotlight has focused on a new form of meningitis caused by the bacteria *Neisseria meningitides* – meningitis C. While much rarer, it can be fatal about 10 per cent of the time. But because it often affects teenagers, we only recommend having your baby vaccinated if there are older children also living in your house. Unfortunately, these vaccines are so new, it is hard to say how effective they are and what side effects they may have.

When protection can be worse than the disease

Perhaps the most contentious question of all involves the negative side effects, including permanent damage or death, due to the vaccination itself. Most commonly, a negative response to a vaccine is a result of a reaction to one or several ingredients in the vaccine, while other cases involve a person's immune response to the infectious agent. However, a baby obviously has a very immature immune system, so is more likely to react than an older child or adult.

Until recently, most vaccines contained a germicidal compound called Thimerosal, which consisted – in part – of mercury. Many vaccines also contain formalin, a 37 per cent solution of formaldehyde, the main ingredient of embalming fluid. Some also contain phenol or ethylene glycol, the main component found in antifreeze. While all of these ingredients are disturbing, Thimerosal is particularly concerning, not only because mercury is a highly toxic element, but also due to the fact that many babies and children are allergic to this compound.

A recent investigation into Thimerosal and the neurological development of children found that the sum total of mercury an average child would receive from normally recommended vaccinations exceeds the US Federal Safety Guidelines for orally ingested mercury, and is in fact correlated with a greater risk for neurodevelopmental disorders.[20] Thankfully, more and more vaccines are being produced without Thimerosal.

But worse still is the vaccine for whooping cough, which accounts for more than half of all reported reactions to vaccinations. Because whooping cough is rarely deadly among well-nourished children, there is a serious question in regard to the benefits of the vaccine in view of its known risks. According to research at the Churchill Hospital in Oxford, England, a baby or child vaccinated against whooping cough is 50 per cent more likely to develop asthma or allergies later in life. This may be because the whooping cough vaccine promotes an abnormally strong immune response to potential allergens such as pollen or gluten, and may disturb early immune programming.

Combination vaccines

While no one yet knows the combined risks of having a number of vaccinations, two of the most common combination vaccinations –

MMR (measles, mumps and rubella) and DPT (diphtheria, pertussis/whooping cough and tetanus) – were thoroughly investigated by the US Centers for Disease Control and Prevention.

In monitoring 500,000 American children after vaccination, thirty-four major side effects were identified, the most common being seizures. Researchers found that the day after a DPT shot, children were three times more likely to have a fit. After the MMR injection, fits were 2.7 times higher after four to seven days and 3.3 times higher after eight to fourteen days.

And that's just seizures. In some cases, DPT reactions have resulted in permanent neurological damage (1 in 30–50,000 children vaccinated) and even death.

MMR is still undoubtedly the most controversial vaccine. Dr Andrew Wakefield's 1998 research study, published in the *Lancet*, first noted a link between the MMR vaccine and developmental disorders, including autism, in a group of children with inflammatory bowel disease. Since then the evidence has been growing. For example, in one survey of 825 parents whose children had symptoms that would classify them as autistic, 55 reported clear signs of regression following the MMR vacccine.

It certainly makes sense to us that a baby or child's immune system is more likely to react to a combination of infectious agents delivered in one package. However, it is probable that reactions are more likely to occur in a baby who has a poor nutritional base, and therefore cannot restore balance after his or her immune system has been forced to react to the threat of an invading organism.

In immune-compromised babies and children, vaccinations may overload their immune systems, resulting in toxic damage to their nervous system and brain. For this reason, more and more parents are seeking out single vaccines instead of combination vaccines.

Alternatives to vaccination

The best alternative to vaccination is to ensure that you and your baby have a fit immune system – and that's what the advice in this book aims to achieve. For the first six months to a year, there is no better way to confer immunity than through breast feeding. Once weaned, you can help to ensure immunity by providing an optimal intake of immune-boosting nutrients.

For example, vitamin A offers protection against measles and probably polio. In underdeveloped countries, deaths from measles have been virtually eliminated with adequate amounts of vitamin A. (See chapter 22 for amounts to supplement.)

Another way to minimise risk in babies, whose immune systems are particularly immature, is to restrict their exposure to large numbers of other potentially infected infants. If possible, we recommend that you avoid placing your child in day care with many other children or involving them in large playgroups, especially in the first couple of years, until their immune systems are much stronger.

If you do choose to give your baby a vaccination, ask your doctor for (1) a list of ingredients in the vaccine, (2) evidence that it works and (3) a list of possible adverse effects. You should also be wary of continuing with vaccinations if your baby has had a bad reaction to a previous vaccine, is currently sick, or if there is any family history of epilepsy, convulsions, neurological disorders, severe allergies or immune system disorders.

Finally, and most importantly, use your common sense. The truth is, we don't have all the answers and don't know the long-term consequences of mass immunisation. In the meantime, gather all the information you can, then let the facts rather than habit or societal pressure guide your decision.

Most common vaccinations and recommendations

Disease	Vaccinate as baby or child	Vaccinate during teenage years	Vaccinate as needed	No need to vaccinate
Measles	X			
Mumps		X		
Chickenpox				X
Rubella		X		
Diphtheria	X			

Disease	Vaccinate as baby or child	Vaccinate during teenage years	Vaccinate as needed	No need to vaccinate
Whooping cough (Pertussis)				X
Tetanus	X			
Polio			X	
Meningitis (Hib)	X	X		
Meningitis C		X		

All vaccines are available privately as separate or single combination vaccines.

Recommended books and websites

The Truth about Vaccinations, Dr Richard Halvorsen, Gibson Square Books 2007.

Are Vaccines Safe and Effective?, Neil Z. Miller, New Atlantean Press 2003.

Immunization – Reality Behind the Myth, Walene James, Greenwood Press 1995.

The Vaccination Bible, Lynne McTaggart, London: HarperCollins 2000.

www.wddty.co.uk – the website for What Doctors Don't Tell You

PART FOUR

OPTIMUM NUTRITION FOR BABIES AND YOUNG CHILDREN

Now that your baby is getting older, you can start introducing them to the wonderful world of food. This is an exciting but also very important time – as your baby grows, sharing a passion and enthusiasm for delicious, nutritious food will lay the foundations for a life of good health. If you've been following the Better Pregnancy Diet, you'll already be eating wholesome food yourself, and this is the best way to educate your child – by being a positive role model.

In this section, we explain:

- When to wean and what food to offer first.

- How to establish healthy eating patterns.

- Which supplements you need to give your child.

- How to tackle food fads and fussiness.

- What to do about crying, sleeping problems and hyperactivity.

- How to keep your baby chemical free.

- How to boost your child's immune system.

꩜

CHAPTER TWENTY

Weaning – When and What

THE QUESTION 'when to wean' is a tricky one, as different people have different opinions. Up until recently, the UK government suggested not before three months, the World Health Organisation recommends waiting until six, and some 'experts' claim that by the time a baby reaches 5.4kg (12lb), breast milk alone can no longer sustain them (which, incidentally, is rubbish). However, as no two babies are the same, there is no definitive answer. But there are some guidelines.

How to know when your baby is ready for solid food

Nature often provides babies with their first teeth at around six months and this seems the most sensible (approximate) time to start introducing some solid food. By this age, your baby's iron reserves will also be running low, so it's important to start introducing some iron-rich solid food to build levels back up again (especially if they were born prematurely). Your baby may actually start to tell you that your milk is not fully meeting their demand – for example if they start feeding every two hours and this goes on for more than five days or if they start waking night after night for a feed when they'd previously been sleeping through. By the time your baby reaches nine months, the protein content of your milk will begin to decline, so it's important that by this stage, they are already getting used to eating solids to meet their additional nutritional needs.

Weaning is a gradual process – not only does your baby need time to get used to solid food, but you also need time to let your milk supply adapt to reduced demand so your breasts don't become painfully engorged. For the first few weeks, you need only introduce a few teaspoons of food at one meal – perhaps lunchtime (or suppertime if your baby is waking in the night) – with breast milk given before and after, and then at all other feeding times.

Your baby will eat very little to start with as he or she has little idea of how to swallow solids (your milk is conveniently delivered to the back of their mouth). Most of what you feed will probably end up all over their face, as in their attempts to swallow, their tongue will come forward and push most of it out again. This is why it's a good idea to start with breast milk to stave off any immediate hunger so they don't become too frustrated.

By weeks three and four, your baby should have got the hang of swallowing, so try increasing the amount of food (maybe three or four teaspoons) and give it in the same way (halfway through feeding) at two meals a day. Continue building, with 'mixed' feeding at three mealtimes, for example, in weeks five and six, moving on to one complete meal with two other mixed feeds in weeks seven and eight, until by the twelfth week, your baby is only having a breast feed last thing at night.

Obviously if your baby is very 'sucky' you may want to continue with breast feeds more often. You can go on supplementing a diet of solid food with your milk for as long as you want – some women choose to carry on for a year, others longer. The immunological properties of breast milk continue to provide both nutrition and protection from illness for as long as your baby continues to suckle.

Keep your baby allergy free

A baby's digestive system is not mature enough to handle solid food much before four months because their digestive tract is still porous and large molecules of protein can pass through before being fully digested. This can trigger an immune response because food anywhere other than the digestive tract is treated as a foreign invader and this can cause an allergy to develop. So, to keep your baby allergy free, breast feed exclusively for at least four months (cow's milk formula is more allergenic than human milk because its protein molecules are much larger).

At the start of weaning, give your baby food that is very easily digested – cooked, puréed vegetables and fruits are a good start. The later that you introduce other foods the less likelihood there is of producing an allergic reaction. We've compiled a list with the least allergenic foods at the top, with guidelines as to when to introduce those foods that are more likely to cause a problem. Omit, too, for as long as possible, any others that you suspect may not suit your baby – for example, because there is a family history of allergy to a certain food or you developed an intolerance while you were pregnant.

Baby's first foods: what and when to introduce while weaning

From 4–6 months

- Vegetables, except tomatoes, potatoes, peppers and aubergines (members of the nightshade family)

- Fruits (except citrus)

- Pulses and beans

- Rice, quinoa, millet and buckwheat

- Fish (preferably organic, wild or deep sea)

From 9 months

- Meat and poultry (preferably organic)
- Oats, corn, barley and rye
- Live yoghurt
- Tomatoes, potatoes, peppers and aubergines
- Eggs
- Soya (i.e. tofu or soya milk)

From 12 months

- Citrus fruits
- Wheat
- Dairy products
- Nuts and seeds (but not peanuts – wait as long as you can before introducing these, and then only organic varieties)

To begin with, introduce only one food each day, make a note of it and watch for any possible reaction. This could be anything from a skin rash or eczema, excessive sleepiness, a runny nose, an ear infection, dark circles under eyes, excessive thirst, over-activity or asthmatic breathing. If you notice anything amiss, stop giving that food and then introduce another once the reaction has died down. You can double-check your observations a few months later when the reaction may have disappeared as the digestive system matures.

Conversely, once you've established a varied mix of foods that cause no reaction, it's then important to vary your child's diet as much as possible, especially with commonly allergenic foods such as wheat, dairy, soya and citrus fruits. Eating the same thing over and over again long term can overtax the system, which can then induce an allergy. But, also, a varied diet will expand your child's desire for a wider range of foods – and this will also ensure they're getting a broader range of nutrients.

Baby's first food

When you start weaning, your baby will still be getting the majority of the protein, fat and carbohydrate they need from your breast milk (which is why, at least initially, you'll find yourself feeding as much as before). So your baby's first foods should be vitamin- and mineral-rich vegetables and fruit – especially those that are good sources of iron (see below). Choose organic if you can, so you are not polluting your baby with residues from artificial fertilisers or pesticides. If a fruit or vegetable can be given raw then leave it raw, for example, bananas, avocados, very ripe William's pears or papaya. Otherwise, steam (to retain more nutrients) or boil in filtered water until soft, then purée with a little of the cooking water until really smooth using a blender or liquidiser. Texture is as important as taste to a baby, so avoid anything slimy or with lumps at this stage.

To start with, make single purées so you can test your baby has no reaction. Try:

- vegetables: carrot, broccoli,* sweet potato, spinach,* kale,* pumpkin or squash, Jerusalem artichoke, leek,* turnip, cauliflower, beetroot, celery, broad beans, avocado, fennel

- fruits: apple, papaya, pear, apricots, kiwi, mixed berries, dried fruit* (i.e. apricots, apples, figs, prunes – but choose unsulphured varieties from your healthfood shop)

When you're ready to mix, good combinations include:

- carrot, spinach and cauliflower

- cauliflower and turnip

- broad beans and cauliflower or carrot and a very little celery

- Jerusalem artichokes and carrot

- peeled courgettes (the skins can be bitter) and fennel

- leek and sweet potato

*These are all good sources of iron, so try to include a few servings of these a week.

- swede, turnip and sweet potato

- avocado and banana

- apple and apricot.

Next, you can start adding brown rice, millet, quinoa (all available as flakes from healthfood shops) or lentil* purée – again, try these foods alone first, then if your baby has no reaction, mix them in with vegetables or fruit. For example, try millet and banana porridge for breakfast or brown rice with carrot and leek for lunch. Just have fun experimenting – there is no limit to the number of combinations you can come up with.

Finally, you can add meat or fish – again preferably organic (i.e. organic chicken) or wild (i.e. wild salmon). Cook it well and purée it, and after first establishing your baby has no reaction, mix with grains and/or vegetables so you start feeding a more balanced meal, for example, cod, sweet potato and broccoli, or salmon, puy lentils and spinach.

To save time and effort, make up enough purée to fill a tray of ice cubes, then spoon in what you've not used and freeze for later (but use within a month or so). One ice-cube-sized portion will provide enough for a meal in the first stages of weaning, then later, you can just use two or more as needed. You can also mix with expressed breast milk to make it taste more like what your baby's used to. However, while convenient, don't be tempted to heat food (or milk) in a microwave. Although it retains nutrient content, it has a negative impact on the immune-protecting properties and can adversely affect your child's blood.[1]

Invariably, there will be times when you have to go out without being able to take food with you. So check out sources of organic baby food jars in your local supermarket or healthfood shop. In the UK, Organix and Hipp use organic ingredients and are free of sugar, additives and preservatives. Or just pack a few pieces of fruit – for example an avocado and a banana – and mash them up as needed.

*These are all good sources of iron, so try to include a few servings of these a week.

The next stage of food discovery

For the first few months of weaning, your baby will only be able to manage finely puréed foods. But by the time they get to about nine months, they'll be ready to explore new textures and types of food.

Nine months

Your baby will now be able to eat 'finger foods' such as raw carrot or apple slices. The gnawing action will also help their teeth come through by acting as an edible teething ring (but watch out for anything that could cause choking). Instead of puréeing, some foods can now be mashed, minced or grated, as your baby will be able to handle small lumps. He or she will also be able to start drinking from a cup, so give water to drink (see page 203).

Twelve months

By now, your baby will probably want to feed him or herself, so provide a plastic spoon or fork and cover the floor under the high chair with a wipe-clean mat. Some foods will still need mashing, but others, such as cooked vegetables or fish, can be eaten in small pieces, and more finger foods such as vegetable or fruit slices and oatcakes can be enjoyed – especially as your baby will still be teething.

Eighteen months

Your baby will now be eating what the rest of the family eats, but watch out for anything too salty or sugary. You can also get them to sit at the table with you if you use a booster seat instead of a high chair.

How much does my baby need?

In the initial stages of weaning, it's easy to follow the feeding pattern established by breast feeding. But later, one of the most common questions parents ask is how much should their baby eat. While some are thinking their babies are not getting enough because they are still not sleeping through the night and do not have rolls of puppy fat, others fear theirs are overfed because they seem to be constantly eating and still have 'chubby' thighs and face. There are a few important points to make here.

First, it is very hard to underfeed a baby if food is made available three times a day. If your baby is not sleeping through the night, this may be due to many reasons, only one of which is hunger. So try giving some extra food at the last meal of the day for a few nights (but don't force it). If it makes no difference, go back to your old feeding patterns. A baby or toddler will know how much food he or she wants. All you need to do is take out the greed element, so don't offer snack foods including extra sweet or salty things packaged in bright, appealing packages. If your child is hungry, a piece of fruit will satisfy them. If they are greedy, only a chocolate biscuit will do.

A baby's natural make-up is to have a certain amount of fat. How much fat your baby has depends on inherited traits, whether he or she is about to have a growth spurt (before a spurt they may well look a little fatter, whereas after they can appear lean), how active they are and also what and how much you are feeding them. On the other hand, if your baby has no rolls of fat and does not have a chubby face, look at other family members first to see if they are also slimly built. If not and your child seems lacking in energy and is sleeping a lot, then they are not getting either enough food or enough of the right kind of nutritious food.

Three main meals a day should be the staple, but these need supplementing with snacks in between to keep your child's energy levels up. You might want to give them some puréed fruit or a breast feed early morning before breakfast, then a mid-morning snack before and a mid-afternoon snack after lunch, with a breast milk feed before bed. Also be sure that you've giving them enough protein.

Does my baby need to drink milk?

For as long as you breast feed, you don't need to supplement your baby's diet with cow's milk. However, once you stop, you will need to ensure your baby gets a good source of calcium. Milk has been marketed for decades as the perfect calcium-rich food, especially for young children. But the key word here is 'marketed'.

We have evolved over millions of years without having any milk after weaning, and still managed to develop strong bones and teeth. There is no evidence that once humans ceased to be nomadic hunter-gatherers and began to cultivate the land, eating grains and keeping animals for meat and milking, their bones got stronger. In fact, the opposite appears to be the case. We appear to have shrunk in size by five or six inches! This, however, is thought to be due to difficulty dealing with grains, more than lack of milk.[2] In many cultures today, milk is still considered food only for babies. So, while milk is widely consumed by our society, we've seen no evidence that it's essential for good health. And as many people develop allergies to it, it's not a good idea for your child to become too reliant on milk – as long as you make sure their diet is rich in other sources of calcium. See the chart on page 196 for the best foods containing calcium.

If you decide you do want to give your child some milk, reduce its allergic potential by rotating cow's milk with goat and sheep's milks plus soya, rice and nut milks (but wait until they are a year old before introducing nut products) – visit your local healthfood shop for a full selection. We ourselves buy a variety and switch between them – using up one carton before opening a different type of milk.

Yoghurt is often better tolerated than milk as the live bacteria that make it predigest a lot of the problematic milk sugars and proteins. Live yoghurt, especially, in which these bacteria remain intact, can help to promote a healthy digestive system. And the calcium in yoghurt is easier to absorb than milk. Goat and sheep's yoghurts are also easy to find in the shops, so again you can have more variety.

The calcium content of foods

Per 100g/100ml	Calcium content (mg)
Cheddar cheese	720
Tahini (sesame seed paste)	680
Sesame seeds	670
Sardines (canned in oil)	550
Almonds	240
Spring greens (raw)	210
Watercress	170
Brazil nuts	170
Kale	150
Tofu (enriched with calcium)	150
Blackstrap molasses (per tablespoon)	150
Whole milk	115

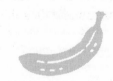

CHAPTER TWENTY-ONE

Optimum Nutrition for a Healthy Baby

I N CHAPTER 9, we explored the building blocks of good nutrition in the context of your diet during pregnancy. While the fundamentals are very similar for a child, some of their nutrient needs are slightly different. For example, young children need relatively more protein and essential fats than adults. Knowing a bit about their special needs will help you optimise their diet, and their health and development.

Protein for growth

Protein makes up 25 per cent of our bodies – we need it to build and repair our skin, hair, nails and all our cells. As your child is growing, their need is greater than that of a fully grown adult. But don't feel this means you have to give them lots of milk, meat and cheese. You see, for the vast majority of adults and children, getting enough protein isn't the problem – it's getting too much. Many of us have 50 to 100 per cent more than we need. After all, the protein content of breast milk is just 1.5 per cent and yet a baby more than doubles its size in just a few months. So in the early stages of weaning, your baby will still get all they need from your breast milk. But when they are relying more on solids, you do need to ensure a regular supply of protein, as dietary sources are rarely as high-quality as breast milk.

Animal versus vegetable

Although animal produce is the primary type of protein in a typical Western diet, gram for gram it's only a marginally better source than nuts and seeds, and is no better than soya, quinoa (a delicious South American grain available from healthfood shops) or rice mixed with pulses. Animal protein is also richer in undesirable saturated fats.

Unlike water-soluble vitamins, which are easily excreted when taken in excess, protein is broken down into by-products (ammonia, uric acid and urea) that are toxic in large amounts and can put stress on the kidneys as they are eliminated. For babies, concentrated protein sources like eggs and meat are hard to tolerate, and should not be introduced in the first nine months of life. Vegetable sources of protein such as lentils and beans, non-gluten grains (e.g. quinoa, millet) and seed vegetables (e.g. broccoli, green beans) contain a higher source of complex carbohydrate and less fat, and are better all round.

Fish is another important source of protein that is easier to digest. Fish is also low in saturated fats and, if you choose oily varieties, high in essential fats. See page 82 for the best fish to choose, as some sources these days are dangerously polluted.

If you do feed your baby meat, try to make sure it's organic so you limit his or her exposure to antibiotics and artificial chemicals or hormones. In chapter 9, on page 91, you will find a table of the best protein sources. The food pyramid on page 204 gives you an idea of how many servings your child needs each day, but as a guide, once your baby is eating three meals a day, include three servings of good-quality protein food such as quinoa, beans or lentils mixed with grains, 'seed' vegetables (i.e. broccoli, corn or peas), organic poultry or lean meat, fish, soya (i.e. tofu) or cheese.

Raising a vegetarian or vegan child

Over three million people in Britain are vegetarian, eating no meat and fish, and a further seven million people avoid all red meat.[3] The number of vegans – eating no animal products, including dairy foods or eggs – is about 0.5 per cent of the population,[4] or 285,000 people. And these numbers are growing. But vegetarianism itself is nothing new – even the ancient Greek mathematician Pythagoras shunned meat in favour of vegetarian foods. And as we've seen, as long as you give your child a good balance of vegetable protein, they won't become deficient. However, you do need to make sure you don't fall into the trap of serving a meal with everything but the meat and no protein alternative. And certain vitamins and minerals are more easily absorbed from animal products – iron, zinc, and vitamins B12 and B6 being the main four. So follow these simple guidelines to provide your child with a nutrient-rich diet.

- To increase absorption of iron from non-meat sources, serve foods containing iron with vitamin-C-rich foods (see chapter 10 for food lists). So, for example, mash a boiled egg with some finely chopped watercress or follow with a berry purée, or serve a good variety of vegetables and fruits that contain both iron and vitamin C (e.g. kale, broccoli, dried fruits).
- To ensure a good supply of zinc, give your child fresh, unsalted seeds to eat (after the age of twelve months) – so sprinkle freshly-ground pumpkin and sunflower seeds over breakfast dishes or add to soups, and spread tahini (sesame seed spread) or almond/cashew butter on oatcakes.
- Boost levels of essential fats with seeds (as above) and add linseeds to your seed mixture, grinding to release the oils. These are excellent for brain and nervous development.
- Soya products are high in protein and calcium (again, introduce them after the age of twelve months) and, as long as your child isn't allergic, include them a few times a week, especially if they are not eating any dairy. See page 105 for other sources of calcium-rich foods.

- Fermented soya products such as tempeh, fortified yeast extracts (but choose low salt) and fortified non-dairy milks are good sources of B12, as are eggs and dairy products for vegetarians. Also include regular sources of B6 – it's found in cabbage, cantaloupe melons, wheatgerm and bran, blackstrap molasses (use to sweeten homemade cakes) and bananas.

- Let weaned vegan babies spend twenty minutes outside in natural sunlight three times a week with their faces and hands exposed so that their skin can synthesise vitamin D. If you live in a sunny climate halve this time and use a high SPF suncream. Non vegans can get vitamin D from dairy products (and fish if you decide to give this to your child).

- As with any diet, we recommend supplementing with extra vitamins and minerals. The key nutrients are B6, B12, iron and zinc – B12 is particularly key for a vegan child. So make sure your supplement contains a good balance of these nutrients (see page 208 for the suggested amounts based on age).

Fats for health

Chapter 8 explains the difference between good and bad fats and shows you how to get the right balance of essential fats in your diet. The same applies for your child.

While you are breast feeding, your baby will get a good source of the Omega 3 fats DHA and AA via your milk (as long as you yourself are) and, if bottle feeding, we suggest supplementing formula milk with cod liver oil (see page 67). These fats are key for healthy nerve and brain development, and a deficiency can mean a lower IQ in later life.

In the first few months of weaning, your breast milk will continue to be your baby's main source of essential fats and, as your baby begins to eat more solids, you can serve oily fish – a rich source of Omega 3 fats (but see page 30 for cautions). After the age of one, we recommend you introduce nuts and seeds – rich in both Omega 3 and 6 fats. See page 84 for daily ground seed formula.

To limit saturated fat, choose lean meats and poultry over red meat and don't give your baby any fried foods or processed foods made with hydrogenated fats (cakes and biscuits that aren't homemade, and some margarines – check the labels).

* As your child becomes less reliant on breast milk, feed oily fish three times a week and, after the age of twelve months, introduce a daily dessertspoon of ground seeds to their diet.

Carbohydrates for energy

Our bodies are designed to run on carbohydrates – we break them down into simple sugars, then 'burn' these to produce energy. As your child is growing, their need to make energy is greater – but growing happens in spurts, so at times they won't seem very hungry, while at others they'll be ravenous.

Because children's need for energy is constant, they need a constant supply. And the best type of fuel is slow burning. So choose wholegrains over refined and include plenty of foods that provide both carbohydrate and protein or fibre (which further slows down energy release), such as lentils, beans, fruits and vegetables, quinoa, brown rice, nuts and seeds.

Fibre is not only essential to regulate energy release, but also to regulate digestive function. Babies may fill four or five nappies a day and, once weaned, your child should still have regular bowel movements that are soft and easy to pass. If you follow the guidelines outlined in the food pyramid and choose wholegrains over refined foods, your child should be getting enough fibre. But as fibre absorbs water, make sure your child is also drinking enough liquid (see page 203).

* Choose wholegrain over refined carbohydrates – so opt for brown rice, millet, quinoa and buckwheat, and avoid anything made with white flour.

* Aim to feed your child four servings of carbohydrates each day – more when they appear hungry. For example, serve oat or millet

201

porridge for breakfast; an oat cake with hummus for a mid-morning snack; quinoa with steamed vegetables (puréed if necessary) for lunch; a sweet potato with salmon and broccoli for supper, followed by homemade rice pudding sweetened with fruit.

Milk and beans: allergy or enzyme deficiency?

Most types of bean (including soya) and pulse contain a type of sugar called amyloglucosidase, which some children and adults find difficult to digest. The consequence is bloating and wind (which is why beans make you fart!), but this is not necessarily an allergy. In the same way that some people find it difficult to digest lactose in milk because they lack the lactase enzyme that breaks this sugar down, so those who experience problems with beans may do so because they lack the enzyme amyloglucosidase. However, in both cases it's possible to supplement these enzymes. See the Resources section for details of suppliers.

Vital vitamins and minerals

In chapter 10, we looked at each different nutrient and what it does for both you and your developing baby. Now your child is born, getting a good supply is still as important and the roles these nutrients played in their early development continue as they grow. The optimum levels for each are illustrated on page 125 and we do suggest you supplement to ensure your child gets what they need. However, the diet is the most important source, so to boost levels of vitamins and minerals:

- Give your child a varied and multicoloured mix of different fruits and vegetables such as red beetroot and plums, orange sweet potatoes and apricots, pale green apples and kiwi, dark green kale and broccoli, blue berries, yellow peppers, etc. Aim for at least six portions a day.

- Where possible, give your child raw fruit or vegetables – as a baby, mashed avocados, bananas and pears, for example, and later as salads, carrot and celery sticks or crunchy apples.

- Certain foods contain a natural substance called oxalic acid and this can impede the absorption of minerals – these include spinach, rocket and rhubarb, so while we don't suggest you avoid these, just don't feed them at every meal. Phytates found in grains can do the same, so again, don't rely on too many grains at every meal – vary the diet and mix and match between rice or wheat with alternatives such as quinoa and millet (available from healthfood shops).

Water for life

Like your body, your child's body is made largely of water, so ensuring a regular supply is essential for cells, organs and tissues to function. The brain, too, is also dependent on water – even mild dehydration can interfere with concentration and cause headaches. While your baby is exclusively breast or bottle fed, they should get all the water they need from your milk or formula. However, as they are weaned on to solids, you will need to give some water to drink.

By around nine months, babies can hold a beaker, so fill it with pure water – filtered and then boiled is the best way to remove the pollutants, as mineral waters can be high in sodium (however, only boil filtered water once, since boiling twice increases its sodium content). But don't wait for your child to ask – by the time we register thirst, we are already dehydrated. A diet rich in fruit and vegetables will also provide water in a very available form, so try to ensure your child eats six or more servings each day. And don't be tempted to give juice – fruit juice is rich in natural sugars but low in fibre (as the flesh and skin have been removed), so can cause a sudden energy surge as well as harming developing teeth. Your child only need drink water or breast milk for the first few years, then have juice diluted with 50 per cent water. By this stage, they will also be used to drinking water and so should continue the habit through life.

- Aim to give your baby between one to two pints of pure water each day – while breast feeding, your milk will provide all they need, but as you start to wean, give your baby a bottle of boiled, filtered water if they are not feeding as much and introduce a feeder cup when they are nine months old.

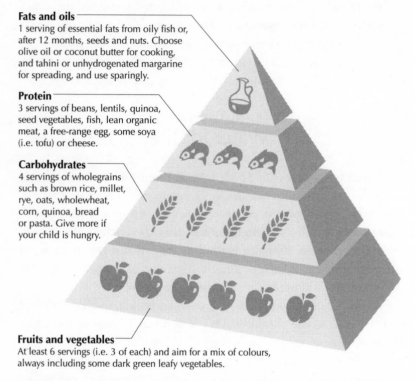

Fats and oils
1 serving of essential fats from oily fish or, after 12 months, seeds and nuts. Choose olive oil or coconut butter for cooking, and tahini or unhydrogenated margarine for spreading, and use sparingly.

Protein
3 servings of beans, lentils, quinoa, seed vegetables, fish, lean organic meat, a free-range egg, some soya (i.e. tofu) or cheese.

Carbohydrates
4 servings of wholegrains such as brown rice, millet, rye, oats, wholewheat, corn, quinoa, bread or pasta. Give more if your child is hungry.

Fruits and vegetables
At least 6 servings (i.e. 3 of each) and aim for a mix of colours, always including some dark green leafy vegetables.

The Food Pyramid

What is a serving?

On page 92, we outline what a serving for an adult is. But when we say to give your baby or child a serving of protein or six portions of fruit or vegetables, how does this translate? For a baby of six to nine months, a serving is approximately one tablespoon; from nine to twelve months, between one and one-and-a-half tablespoons; then once he or she gets past a year, about two tablespoons of cooked food, or a quarter of an apple or carrot. However, there is no exact science here – a serving is really just a unit that helps you measure the proportion of food your child eats in a day so you can achieve a balanced diet.

CHAPTER TWENTY-TWO

Supplements for Super Kids

CCORDING TO Dr Roger Williams, a pioneer in optimum
nutrition who helped discover folic acid and vitamin B5,
'The greatest hope for increasing [health and] lifespan can be
offered if nutrition – from the time of pre-natal development up to
old age – is continuously of the highest quality.' Although a varied
and nutritious diet is the key foundation to good health, as we've
demonstrated in chapter 12, even the best diets can fail to provide
appropriate levels of all the nutrients we need. And for some essential nutrients, such as folic acid, supplements have been proven to be
twice as effective in raising body levels and improving body chemistry than the same amount in food.[5]

As children can sometimes be picky eaters (not to mention the
logistical challenge of providing a day's meals perfectly balanced in
every nutrient), supplementing their diet is the most reliable way to
ensure they get appropriate levels of all the vitamins and minerals they
need to be optimally nourished. Calcium and vitamin D are key for
bone development as around 45 per cent of adult bone mass is formed
before eight years of age. B vitamins are essential for energy production and a healthy immune system. Zinc is imperative for growth, iron
for the formation of red blood and the transport of oxygen to the body
cells. There is not one vitamin or mineral that isn't still essential for

good health. If they miss out, just a small deficiency in any nutrient can have a serious impact for growing children.

The age to start supplementing

If you've followed the Supplement Plan during your pregnancy and continued with the supplements recommended while breast feeding, your baby's food source has already been indirectly supplemented. Moving on to giving babies supplements directly is not a recommendation made only by nutritionists or complementary therapists – the UK government provides vitamin drops free of charge for young children up to the age of five via your family doctor.

However, these drops provide only very basic levels of supplementation and exclude many key vitamins and minerals. Especially important for a growing child are vitamin A to build up strong membranes less permeable to infection; vitamin D to aid the absorption of calcium; B vitamins and vitamin C involved in brain development, making energy and a healthy immune system; calcium and magnesium for healthy bones; zinc to maintain the integrity of RNA and DNA (our genetic blueprint) and assist in growth; essential fatty acids because these get incorporated into every cell – especially brain cells; and also iron, chromium, selenium and manganese.

We recommend you start supplementing your child's diet when they begin to rely more on solid food rather than breast milk for their main source of nutrients. This is usually at around the age of six to nine months. The ideal daily supplement programme we recommend from weaning to age eleven is shown in the chart on page 208.

The ideal daily supplement programme

Age Nutrient	Less than 1	1	2	3–4	5–6	7–8	9–11
Vitamins							
A (retinol)	500mcg	600	700	800	1,000	1,500	2,000
D	1mcg	1.25	1.5	1.75	2.25	2.5	2.5
E	13mg	13	17	20	23	30	40
C	100mg	100	200	300	400	500	600
B1 (thiamine)	5mg	5	6	8	12	16	20
B2 (riboflavin)	5 mg	5	6	8	12	16	20
B3 (niacin)	7mg	10	14	16	18	20	22
B5 (pantothenic acid)	10mg	10	15	20	25	30	35
B6 (pyridoxine)	5mg	5	7	10	12	16	20
B12	5mcg	6	7	8	9	10	10
Folic acid	100mcg	100	120	140	160	180	200
Biotin	30mcg	40	50	60	70	80	90
Minerals							
Calcium	150mg	160	170	180	190	200	210
Magnesium	50mg	60	70	80	90	100	110
Iron	4mg	5	6	7	8	9	10
Zinc	4mg	5	6	7	8	9	10
Manganese	300mcg	300	350	400	500	700	1,000
Iodine	50mcg	75	100	125	150	175	200
Chromium	15mcg	17	20	23	25	27	30
Selenium	10mcg	15	20	25	28	30	35
GLA	50	65	80	95	110	135	150
EPA	100	150	200	250	300	350	400
DHA	100	125	150	175	200	225	250

Choosing the right supplements

Many companies formulate single multivitamin and mineral supplements that incorporate all the necessary nutrients especially for children (see Resources on page 250). The chart provided in this chapter will give you a guideline as to the levels of nutrients to look for. You can choose chewable (crushable in the early stages) or liquid formulas, depending on your (or your child's) preferences. And you should ideally give your child his or her supplement with breakfast, but certainly not last thing at night as the B vitamins can have a mild stimulatory effect. Children also tend to be more susceptible to vitamin toxicity than adults, and while the doses listed are well within any potentially toxic limits for even the most sensitive child, don't be tempted to give more than the recommended levels unless under the direction and supervision of a nutritional therapist.

Essential fats to boost IQ

As long as your child is eating oily fish three times a week and a daily portion of seeds (see page 84), then they should be getting a good level of essential fats to help their brains develop and boost IQ. However, if they don't eat fish or don't have seeds every day, then we recommend you supplement their diet with an essential fatty acid (EFA) formula. Look for one that contains both GLA (Omega 6) and DHA and EPA, which are the most important Omega 3 fats for development (see the Resources section for details). The chart opposite gives you the rough quantities to aim for in a supplement, assuming your child is receiving the same again from seeds and the occasional fish.

CHAPTER TWENTY-THREE

Food Fads and Fussiness

'MY CHILD WILL only eat chocolate yoghurt.' 'My child will only eat spaghetti hoops and baked beans.' 'My child will only eat potatoes, carrots and sausages.' Anyone who has anything to do with children will recognise these phrases well. However, there are some simple ways to deal with food fads and fussiness so they don't compromise your child's health (or your sanity!).

Prevention is better than cure

First, if you do not have chocolate yoghurt, spaghetti hoops, fizzy drinks or whatever other junk food your child decides they want to eat in the house, then you will never get into this situation as the option isn't there. If possible, try to find healthy alternatives – for example, serve carob powder added to live yoghurt, wholewheat spaghetti with homemade tomato sauce or orange juice mixed with sparkling water. But if your child still refuses to eat anything but their beloved food, then just wait it out.

Taking the emotion out of mealtimes can also help. The majority of food fads are emotionally driven – they are often vehicles for your child to get attention or assert their independence. So the fewer emotions you display at mealtimes, the better. For example, try not to give out loads of praise for an empty bowl, and don't appear too hurt when your lovingly prepared vegetable casserole goes uneaten.

From the very start, eating should be a matter of satisfying appetite, not something your child does for mummy or something they do tidily or even for starving people. So, let your child's appetite lead their eating, not your desire to feed them. If they want more food one day, give it to them – they could be preparing for a growth spurt. Equally, if their hunger wanes the next day, don't force feed them. They may be unwell or just tired.

Eating should also be an independent thing that your child does for him or herself as soon as possible using spoon or hands, whichever is easier – and preferably (for their enjoyment) messier. So don't be too tough too soon on your child's manners. Let them learn to enjoy food first, and get tidy later.

Dealing with an unwilling eater

If your child doesn't have much of an appetite or is a picky eater, first assess whether the food you are giving them is attractive and appetising. Also, are you offering an interesting variety of meals? Many families rotate six or seven dishes every week and mealtimes can therefore become boring or predictable. If your child refuses whole food groups, for example vegetables, check that you are serving an appealing selection of colours, tastes and textures. A rainbow-coloured stir-fry is more likely to whet their appetites than over-cooked carrots or limp-looking beans. You can also up your child's nutrient intake by means of subterfuge: add grated or mashed vegetables to mince, casseroles, homemade burgers, pasta sauces and soups.

And if your child takes a temporary dislike to something, don't push it; it is far better to have two weeks without eggs than a whole lifetime. Just reintroduce the food again after a short absence and see what happens.

Sometimes it's the other extreme and your child becomes fixated on only eating their favourite foods over and over. But even if these appear limited, as long as the foods are providing a balance of nutrients, don't be too concerned.

Finally, if you are offering interesting and varied food and they still don't want to eat, check their zinc status – as well as poor appetite, do they also have white marks on more than two finger-nails, any stretch marks on the skin, and a poor immune system, or appear listless or depressed? If so, supplement their diet with a multivitamin and mineral formula containing zinc (see page 110).

Helpful strategies for healthy eaters

Manage their choices

It will be a few years before your child has the complete capability to make a choice between, say, risotto or pasta. But while a toddler will not understand if you say, 'What do you want for lunch today?' they may respond if you hold up a banana and a pear and say 'Do you want a banana or a pear?'

Research by the British Food Council shows that children are more willing to eat food they themselves have chosen. So while you need to keep this simple so as not to overwhelm or encourage fussiness initially, as your child grows, you can involve them more. For example, ask them to pick out some fruit and vegetables in the supermarket or get them involved in preparing meals.

Snacks and rewards

While snacks are important for providing a regular source of energy, too many may prevent your child eating proper meals. If this appears to be happening, do not give interesting foods as snacks. If a toddler is really hungry in between meals he or she will happily eat a carrot stick or an oatcake if that's all that's on offer. Drinking lots of milk can also dampen appetite, as it's a food and so is much more filling than a glass of water or diluted fruit juice.

Be careful, too, of rewarding or comforting your child with food – this can lay down emotional patterns that may later encourage them to comfort eat when faced with a difficult situation, which, in the long term, can lead to obesity.

Home versus the outside world

While you can provide your child with healthy food at home, keeping this up when they visit friends, go to parties or eat out can be difficult. But as long as the majority of their diet is nutritious, the occasional burger, drink of cola, packet of crisps or chocolate ice cream won't cause any harm. And if you explain that there's one way of eating at home and another way elsewhere, you can help your child associate these 'treats' with special occasions and not pester you for them all the time. However, it's wise not to make a big issue of this or your child will begin to see certain foods as 'forbidden', which will only enhance their appeal.

When you eat out in restaurants, you don't have to order food from the children's menu if all it offers is fried and processed choices (nuggets and chips, etc.). Order an adult starter or share a main dish with your child, or ask to substitute the chips for a steamed vegetable or a salad. Also, ask for diluted fruit juices instead of fizzy drinks.

☙

CHAPTER TWENTY-FOUR

Crying, Sleeping and Hyperactivity

O F ALL THE things that seem to distress new mothers (and fathers) most, a child who doesn't sleep or who cries all the time seems to come top of the list, followed by overly active or aggressive behaviour. Any one of these is enough to wear down the resolve of even the strongest parent. But what causes these problems and what can be done?

Biochemical imbalances brought about by poor nutrition, food allergy or toxicity can all cause behavioural problems. But before exploring these, it's important to first consider the basics. A baby that cries all the time, for example, may be in severe pain because they have colic (see page 171 for signs and treatment). Or they may just want to be picked up and cuddled.

If your baby's birth was traumatic or very quick, their skull may have been compressed in such a way that the sutures became very subtly misaligned, which can cause lasting discomfort. So if you suspect this may be a factor, it's worth finding a cranial osteopath. A cranial osteopath holds the baby's head very gently and allows the different cranial plates to realign with a very subtle touch, so they can develop properly. A few sessions of cranial osteopathy can be very helpful. (See the Resources section for details.)

Not sleeping through the night?

Children can wake up for lots of reasons – they may be scared or lonely, feel unwell, or be too hot, too cold or have an uncomfortable wet nappy. But they may also be hungry, especially if they wake at the same time each night. If this is the case, then you have a number of options. If they are still breast or bottle fed, you could wake them up before you go to bed and give them a feed – this will then hopefully sustain them through the rest of the night. If they are eating solids, then give them a healthy snack just before they go to bed. Also make sure the food they are getting provides a stable source of energy that won't lead to 'blood sugar lows' (see page 220 for more on this) in the middle of the night.

Active or hyperactive?

Many children are incredibly active and this can be a good sign of intelligence and natural curiosity, even if it leaves the parents exhausted. Children can also go through difficult stages of development where they may have interrupted sleep or throw tantrums (during the 'terrible twos' for example). But a hyperactive child is quite different. Classically, a hyperactive child is disorganised and has difficulty concentrating. Attention span is very short, often only a few seconds, so the child will change what he or she is doing all the time, and the child's mood is equally changeable.

'He's really such a nice child but sometimes he becomes so aggressive, literally biting or hitting me.' This sort of statement describes the rapid mood swings so often seen in hyperactive children. Their sleep is often disturbed and they may also cry a lot. These signs can occur from birth, and before, according to a recent study, which found that excessive 'foetal kicking' during pregnancy is associated with high risk for hyperactive symptoms.

The good news is that, more often than not, hyperactive children have one or more nutritional imbalance that, once identified and corrected, can dramatically improve their energy, focus, concentration and behaviour.

Is your child hyperactive?

It can be difficult to draw the line between the behaviour of a child that is within the normal limits of high energy and abnormally active behaviour. This checklist will help you determine where your child's behaviour falls, although if your child is very young, then many characteristics won't yet apply. Where you can, assess each characteristic and score 2 if a symptom is severe, 1 if moderate and 0 if not present.

Overactive	Doesn't finish projects
Fidgets	Wears out toys, furniture, etc.
Can't sit still at meals	Doesn't stay with games
Talks too much	Doesn't follow directions
Clumsy	Fights with other children
Unpredictable	Teases
Doesn't respond to discipline	Destructive
Speech problems	Temper tantrums
Doesn't listen to whole story	Defiant
Hard to get to bed	Irritable
Reckless	Unpopular with peers
Impatient	Tells lies
Accident prone	Bed wetter

A score below 12 is normal. Higher scores indicate your child may benefit from the nutritional strategies outlined in this chapter.

Vitamin and mineral supplements to help regulate moods

Studies have shown that behavioural problems diminish significantly when children are given nutritional supplements. In one study by Dr Abram Hoffer, a pioneer in optimum nutrition, large doses of vitamin

C and B3 significantly improved the behaviour of thirty-two out of thirty-three hyperactive children.[6] Other studies have revealed that children may be deficient in zinc or magnesium, both of which can produce symptoms associated with hyperactivity. The symptoms of magnesium deficiency, for example, are excessive fidgeting, anxiety, restlessness, coordination problems and learning difficulties in the presence of a normal IQ. To ensure your child isn't deficient, follow the recommendations for supplements given in chapter 22.

EFAs to reduce symptoms of hyperactivity

Many hyperactive children have symptoms of essential fatty acid (EFA) deficiency, such as excessive thirst, dry skin, eczema and asthma. It is also interesting that boys, who have a much higher EFA requirement than girls, are more commonly affected: four out of five hyperactive children are male. Researchers have theorised that these children may be deficient in EFAs, not just because they have inadequate dietary intake (though this is not uncommon), but rather because their need is higher, because they absorb them poorly or they are not able to convert them well into substances called prostaglandins that help the brain communicate.[7]

It is of interest then that EFA conversion to prostaglandins can be inhibited by most of the foods that cause symptoms in hyperactive children, such as wheat and dairy foods. Conversion is also hindered by deficiencies of the various vitamins and minerals needed to make these conversions happen, including vitamins B3, B6, C, biotin, zinc and magnesium.

If your child is not getting a good dietary source of omega 3 EFAs, add to their diet some oily fish (e.g. organic salmon, sardines, fresh not canned tuna, mackerel) and seeds such as flax, hemp, sunflower and pumpkin or their cold-pressed oils. Also consider eliminating wheat products and dairy products, as well as supplementing the nutrients needed for this conversion via a good multivitamin and mineral formula.

Eliminating brain pollutants

As well as a deficiency in key nutrients, an excess of anti-nutrients can induce behavioural problems. Top of the list is lead, which produces symptoms of aggression, and poor impulse control and attention span. This is more likely to occur in inner city children, especially in parts of the world where lead in petrol is still allowed. Another is excess copper, generally from water pipes in new houses or soft water areas, which is found in some hyperactive children. Studies have also revealed a link between high aluminium and hyperactivity. Many toxic elements deplete the body of essential nutrients, for example zinc, and may contribute to nutritional deficiencies. Conversely, they can accumulate if a child is zinc deficient. If improving the diet doesn't appear to help your child, a hair mineral analysis can check for heavy metal intoxication. This can be arranged via a nutritional therapist (see the Resources section), who can then work to reduce toxicity and restore a healthy mineral balance.

Allergies and behaviour problems

Of all the avenues so far researched, the link between behavioural problems and allergy is the most established and worthy of pursuit in any child displaying hyperactive behaviour or unexplained mood swings.

A study by Dr Joseph Bellanti of Georgetown University in Washington DC found that hyperactive children are seven times more likely to have food allergies than other children. According to his research, 56 per cent of hyperactive children aged between seven and ten tested positive for food allergies, compared to less than 8 per cent of 'normal' children. A separate investigation by the Hyperactive Children Support Group found that 89 per cent of children with Attention Deficit Hyperactivity Disorder (ADHD – an official name for hyperactivity) reacted to food colourings, 72 per cent to flavourings, 60 per cent to MSG, 45 per cent to all synthetic additives, 50 per cent to cow's milk,

60 per cent to chocolate and 40 per cent to orange.[8] For more on food additives, read chapter 25.

Other substances often found to induce behavioural changes are wheat, dairy, corn, yeast, soya, peanuts and eggs.[9] Associated symptoms that are strongly linked to allergy include nasal problems and excessive mucus, ear infections, facial swelling and discoloration around the eyes, tonsillitis, digestive problems, bad breath, eczema, asthma, headaches and bed-wetting. It's relatively simple to identify foods that may be causing or aggravating symptoms by excluding them for two weeks before a carefully observed reintroduction (for more on this, read chapter 7).

Up to 90 per cent of hyperactive children benefit from eliminating foods that contain artificial colours, flavours and preservatives, processed and manufactured foods, and 'culprit' foods identified by either an exclusion diet or blood test.[10] Some have also reported success with the Feingold diet, which involves removing not only all artificial additives but also foods that naturally contain compounds called salicylates. Researchers at the University of Sydney, Australia found that of eighty-six children with ADHD, 75 per cent reacted adversely to foods containing salicylates.[11] These include prunes, raisins, raspberries, almonds, apricots, canned cherries, blackcurrants, oranges, strawberries, grapes, tomato sauce, plums, cucumbers and Granny Smith apples. As the list is very long and contains many otherwise nutritious foods this should be considered only as a secondary course of action, and must be carefully planned and monitored by a nutritional therapist to ensure adequate nutritional intake.

Understanding how a low salicylate diet helps hyperactive children offers us an alternative, however. Salicylates inhibit the conversion and utilisation of essential fatty acids, which we know from the discussion above to be essential for proper brain function and are often low in hyperactive children. So instead of avoiding the inhibitor (salicylates), it may be sufficient to increase the supply of EFAs, which has indeed been shown to help. See chapter 22 for more on EFA supplements.

No sugar thanks, I'm sweet enough already

A diet high in refined carbohydrates is not good for anyone, and many parents believe that eating sweets promotes hyperactivity and aggression in their children. In contrast, some recent research has suggested that sugar itself is not to blame for hyperactivity, and can even have a calming effect on certain individuals. Yet dietary studies do consistently reveal that hyperactive children have higher sugar consumption than other children.[12] It seems then that reactions to sugar are not due to allergy as such, but to a craving brought on by low blood sugar levels (or hypoglycaemia).

Other research has confirmed that the problem is not sugar itself but the forms in which it comes, the absence of a well-balanced diet overall and abnormal glucose metabolism. A study of 265 hyperactive children found that more than three-quarters displayed abnormal glucose tolerance.[13] As the main fuel for the brain and body, when blood glucose levels fluctuate wildly all day on a roller-coaster ride of refined carbohydrates, sweets, chocolate, fizzy drinks, juices and little or no fibre to slow the glucose absorption, it is not surprising that levels of activity, concentration, focus and behaviour will also fluctuate. The calming effect sometimes observed after sugar consumption may well be the initial normalisation of blood sugar from a hypoglycaemic state during which the brain and cognitive functions controlling behaviour were starved of fuel.

Our advice then is not to give your child any form of refined sugar or any foods that contain it. Instead, give wholefoods and complex carbohydrates (brown rice and other whole grains, oats, lentils, beans, quinoa and vegetables) throughout the day. Carbohydrates should always be balanced with protein (half as much protein as carbohydrates at every meal and snack) to improve glucose tolerance, for example nuts with fruit or fish with rice.

In summary, if your child is not sleeping, or is crying or hyperactive:

- **Follow** the guidelines in this book to feed your child plenty of nutrient-rich foods and limit processed, sugary or nutrient-depleted foods.

- **Supplement** your child's diet with a good multivitamin and mineral formula.

- **Boost** levels of essential fats – give your child oily fish a few times a week (but see page 118 for cautions) and incorporate fresh seeds and cold-pressed seed oils into their daily diet.

- **Balance** blood sugar by providing regular meals and snacks with a 50/50 mix of carbohydrate and protein.

- **Eliminate** chemical food additives.

- **Check** for other potential allergens such as wheat, dairy, chocolate, oranges and eggs (see chapter 7 for more on this).

- **If** you are still experiencing problems, visit a nutritional therapist who can arrange a hair mineral analysis to test for heavy metal toxicity.

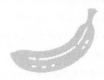

CHAPTER TWENTY-FIVE

❦

Keeping Your Baby Chemical Free

IN THE LAST ten years over 3,000 man-made chemicals have been incorporated into the food we eat. Some have taken the place of natural foods, others are added to foods to make them look more appealing, taste better and/or last longer. Their use has become so widespread that certain foods on the supermarket shelf are completely unrecognisable from their list of ingredients. For example, can you guess what this is?

Ingredients: sugar, starch, salt, hydrogenated vegetable oil, whey powder, lactose, caseinate, gelling agents (E410, E407, E340), potassium chloride, adipic acid, acidity regulator (E336), stabiliser (E446), artificial sweetener (sodium saccharin), colours (E102, E110, E132, E123, E160A), flavourings, emulsifiers (E477, E322), preservative (E202), and antioxidant (E320).

In case you can't guess (and let's face it, who but the 'food' scientist who created it can?), this is a popular brand of banana and tropical fruit flavoured trifle!

So common has the use of food additives become that each one of us inadvertently eats around 5kg of these chemicals each year. Foods aimed at children, in particular, are packed with colourings and flavourings, with the UK Food Commission estimating that 40 per cent of foods and drinks designed for young consumers contain additives. But although they are 'permitted', are these chemicals really safe for our children and us?

Food additives and behavioural problems

As we've already seen, food additives can cause hyperactive behaviour. According to new government research, the use of food colourings in many popular children's foods can trigger temper tantrums and disruptive behaviour in toddlers. Scientists at the UK's Asthma and Allergy Research Centre, working on behalf of the Food Standards Agency, concluded that: 'Significant changes in children's hyperactive behaviour could be produced by the removal of colourings and additives from their diet.' They also suggested that their avoidance would benefit all children – 'not just for those already showing hyperactive behaviour or who are at risk of allergic reactions.'

Colourings as 'anti-nutrients'

The yellow food colouring tartrazine (E102) is the best known of many chemical additives linked to allergies and hyperactive behaviour. But how does it trigger such reactions? One theory is that it acts as an anti-nutrient, depleting the body's stores of beneficial nutrients. In one study that found emotional and behavioural changes in every child who consumed tartrazine, researchers noted that the additive decreased blood levels of zinc by increasing the amount of zinc excreted in the urine.[14] Four out of the ten children in the study also had severe reactions, three developing eczema or asthma within forty-five minutes of ingestion.

This is the first of hundreds of food chemicals to be tested in this way and, of course, it begs the question as to what safety criterion a chemical must meet before being allowed to enter the food chain. Or are new chemicals simply innocent until proven guilty? The legislation on 'novel foods' (created to enhance health) is becoming more stringent, yet the concept of testing for anti-nutrient effects is not on the checklist.

Cracking the 'E' code

As a result of European Union legislation, all food additives are allocated an 'E' number. For manufacturers, this means there's no need to put long lists of chemical-sounding ingredients on their products (just long lists of E numbers), if they choose to use them. For us members of the public, it means it's easier to understand what's in the food we buy. But you need to know how to crack the E numbers code. The first thing to understand is that different types of additive form different E number series. Here are the main categories:

Colours	E100	to	E180
Preservatives	E200	to	E290
Antioxidants	E300	to	E321
Emulsifiers	E322	to	E494
Sweeteners	E420	to	E421
Mineral hydrocarbons	E905	to	E907
Modified starches	E1400	to	E1442

Next you need to decide if you really need any of these. Let's concern ourselves with the first four categories. Colours are added to make our food look good. Of course, if you don't mind eating peas that don't glow in the dark and can accept that smoked haddock isn't naturally bright yellow, then it is best to avoid all food colourings. Except two. E101 is vitamin B2. And E160 is vitamin A. These colouring agents are actually good for you.

Preservatives prevent the growth of micro-organisms like mould. Often the effects of mould are far worse than the effects of preservatives. However, if you can buy food fresh that's the best. It's a matter of choice. Sausages, for example, contain nitrates (E250–E252) to prevent some very dangerous micro-organisms. But the more nitrates you eat, the more you risk forming nitrosamines, which are potent cancer-producing chemicals. No preservatives are actually good for you.

Antioxidants stop food becoming rancid. This is most important for fats and oils. Nature equips foods with antioxidants. Seeds, high in oils, are also high in vitamin E. Vitamin E is a good antioxidant. Its E numbers are E306, E307, E308 and E309. Another natural antioxidant is vitamin C. Its E numbers are E300, E301, E302, E303 and E304. Other antioxidants, such as BHA (E320) and BHT (E321) are of dubious safety.

Emulsifiers help to bind and emulsify sauces. It's the lecithin in egg that makes mayonnaise what it is. Lecithin is E322. Other emulsifiers, like the polyphosphates, E450, are there so that more water can be added to meats, increasing the manufacturer's profits. These are therefore unnecessary.

Additives – good and bad

To help guide you through the maze of E numbers, we've compiled a list of the good and the bad for the main food additive categories. Photocopy this list and then, when shopping, let it guide your food choices. Our advice is to feel good about the 'goods', actively avoid the 'bads' and cut down on any not listed here (although beware: new E numbers are created all the time and so may be even worse for your health!).

Colours (E100–E180)

Good		Bad	
E101	Riboflavin	E102	Tartrazine
E160	Carotene	E104–E142	Mainly coal tar or azo dyes
		E150	Caramel
		E151–E155	Coal tar dyes
		E173	Aluminium
		E174	Silver

Preservatives (E200–E290)

Good		Bad	
		E200–E203	Sorbates
		E210–E219	Benzoates
		E220–E227	Sulphur/sulphites
		E230–E249	Misc.
		E250–E252	Nitrates
		E262	Diacetate
		E281–E283	Propionates
		E290	Carbon dioxide

Antioxidants (E300–E321)

Good		Bad	
E300–E304	Ascorbates	E310–E312	Gallates
E306–E309	Tocopherols	E320	BRA
		E321	BHT

Emulsifiers, stabilisers and others (E322–E925)

Good		Bad	
E322	Lecithin	E385	EDTA
E375	Nicotinic acid	E407	Carrageenan
E440	Pectin	E513	Sulphuric acid
		E525	Potassium hydroxide
		E535	Sodium ferrocyanide
		E541	Sodium aluminium phosphate
		E631	Sodium inositate
		E621	Monosodium glutamate
		E635	Sodium ribonucleotide
		E905	Mineral hydrocarbons
		E924	Potassium bromate
		E925	Chlorine

❦

CHAPTER TWENTY-SIX

Boosting Your Child's Immune System

ONCE YOUR CHILD starts mixing with other children, they will also be socialising with a whole host of new germs that will test their immune system. Many parents complain that their toddlers have a permanent cold, cough or runny nose. But you can help to strengthen your child's immune system with the right nutritional support, making them less prone to developing infections in the first place and increasing their chances of a speedy recovery when they do succumb.

Immune-boosting nutrients

Nature has packaged a range of special immune-boosting substances to help us fight off bugs and viruses and manage the damage caused to our bodies by pollution, environmental toxins and the everyday biochemical processes of life. These are covered in chapter 7 and are the same for your child as they are for you.

So, once you start to wean, you can feed your child antioxidant-rich foods such as sweet potatoes and carrots (vitamin A), berries, kiwi fruit and green leafy vegetables (vitamin C), avocados (vitamin E), fish (zinc) and broccoli (selenium). Ensuring your child eats a varied diet will also ensure he or she is getting a wide range of nutrients – not just vitamins and minerals, but also powerful immune-boosting 'phyto-chemicals', such as flavonoids found in berries and lypocene in toma-toes. Giving plenty of water will help to flush out any toxins and prevent your child becoming dehydrated, which can prevent his or her body functioning effectively.

Your breast milk is also rich in antibodies, which helps your baby fend off infections and boosts their immune system, so continue feed-ing (even if it's only last thing at night) for as long as you can.

However, even with a healthy diet, plenty of water and breast milk, your child will still succumb to infections as this is a vital process to help them build up natural immunity. So when they do fall ill, what can you do to help them recover as quickly as possible?

Infection fighters

A key weapon in the immune-supporting nutritional arsenal is vita-min C. This is both antiviral and antibacterial and boosts production of white blood cells, which are vital soldiers in the body's immune army. If your child has a cold, sore throat, viral infection or the flu, stir vitamin C powder into a glass of water, diluted juice or vegetable/fruit purée and give it four to six times a day until they are well (and then gradually reduce the dose over a few days). For doses, see the chart on page 208, but use the recommended daily amount as a guide to each single dose (i.e. if they are one, give them 100mg four to six times a day). If your child develops loose bowels (a possible side effect), decrease the dose slightly.

You can also get sublingual zinc, or zinc drops, which again help to fight an infection. Don't give your child more zinc than the maximum daily amount recommended for their age. Both vitamin C and zinc are great for kids of any age.

Dairy, meat and eggs can be very mucus making, so if your child is suffering with a streaming nose or chesty cough, stop giving them these foods until they make a compete recovery. If your child has a perma-nent runny nose, then suspect a dairy allergy – see chapter 7 for details.

See also chapter 18 for suggestions to treat other common ailments (colic, constipation and eczema).

Say no to sugar

Sugar suppresses our immune systems. One study found that participants had a 50 per cent reduction in the activity of white blood cells (vital soldiers in the immune army) for five hours or more after ingesting a sugar solution.[15] Our advice is to avoid giving your child any sugar at all, although there are obviously times when this won't be possible. However, if they are unwell or surrounded by other sick children (for example if the gastric flu is going round their nursery), cut out all sugar and give them antioxidant-rich fresh fruit, or treats/desserts sweetened with honey or molasses (see pages 238–40 for some suggestions of these).

Getting physical

Research shows that exercise improves immunity (as well as mood) and prevents diseases such as obesity and diabetes. A healthy child will naturally be full of energy with a desire to be active, so channel this with daily activities such as swimming, walking, dancing or playing games such as chase, throwing a ball or hide and seek. Having an outlet for their energy will also help your child to sleep better.

What about antibiotics?

From time to time, antibiotics are essential to save life. The problem is that with overuse, bacteria are developing resistance and there now exist certain strains that are resistant to even the strongest antibiotics. They also kill off healthy bacteria, so causing an imbalance in the delicate gut flora. Long term this can lead to digestive problems and food allergies, and it has even been linked with attention deficit hyperactivity disorder (ADHD). In a study comparing children with ADHD to those without, Dr Neil Ward of the University of Surrey found that a significantly higher percentage of the hyperactive children had taken several courses of antibiotics in early childhood.[16] Further investigations revealed that children who had had three or more antibiotic courses before the age of three also had significantly lower levels of the essential minerals zinc, calcium, chromium and selenium.[17] Also, children given antibiotics for ear infections triple their chances of another ear infection, according to research published in the *Lancet* medical journal.

So, our advice is to only give your child a course of antibiotics if they are really necessary (i.e. not for a common cold). If you find they are getting repeated infections, rather than resorting to repeated courses of antibiotics, visit a nutritional consultant who can get to the root cause of the problem. When your child does need antibiotics, you can replenish good bacteria with 'probiotics' (see below for more on this). Start supplementing as soon as your child begins taking the antibiotics and continue for a week after the course has finished to restore a healthy balance of gut bacteria.

Probiotics boost immunity

Around 2kg (4lb) of an adult's body weight comes from bacteria that live in their digestive tract. These bacteria total around 100 trillion – that's more than the total number of cells in your body! The right kinds of bacteria are our friends and are known as 'intestinal flora' or probiotics.

Although your baby is born with a sterile gut, intestinal bacteria start to colonise immediately. While not all are 'friendly', as long as your baby has enough of the health-promoting varieties, then any bad bacteria are kept in check and are less likely to cause any problems. There are many other benefits of having a healthy population of beneficial bacteria:

- They make vitamins including vitamins B1, B2, B3, B5, B6, B12, biotin, A and K.

- They fight infections and have been shown to halve recovery time from diarrhoea, prevent overgrowth of salmonella and *E. coli* (the bacteria responsible for many cases of food poisoning), *Helicobacter pylori* and *Candida albicans*.

- They boost immunity by increasing the number of immune cells.

- They promote other 'good' bacteria while reducing 'bad' bacteria. *Lactobacillus acidophilus* supplementation, for instance, has been shown to promote the beneficial Bifidobacteria and inhibit disease-producing microbes.[18]

- They are anti-allergy and have been shown to help reduce chances of developing food allergies and reduce inflammatory reactions during allergic reactions by lessening the response in the gut to allergenic foods.[19]

There are many different strains of 'friendly' bacteria – some of which actually live in the gut, while others simply 'pass through' and are useful while they're there. Here are some of the different types that are most important for children:

The principal friendly bacteria in a child's digestive tract

RESIDENT	*B. infantis*
	B. bifidum
	B. bacterium
	L. acidophilus
PASSING THROUGH	*L. bulgaricus*
	S. thermophilus

Key: B. = *Bifidobacteria*; L. = *Lactobacillus*; S. = *Streptococcus*

Those that are resident, sometimes called 'human strain', are usually more powerful at fighting infection because they multiply and colonise the digestive tract. Others are available in fermented foods such as yoghurt, miso and sauerkraut, and these bacteria will hang around for a week or so doing good work. They, like the other beneficial bacteria, can make vitamins as well as turning lactose, the main sugar in milk, into lactic acid. This makes the digestive tract slightly more acidic, which inhibits disease-causing microbes from multiplying.

Promoting healthy bacteria

Include fermented foods in your child's diet to promote healthy intestinal flora. You could choose:

* yoghurt, cottage cheese, kefir (from dairy produce)

* sauerkraut, pickles (from vegetables)

* miso, tofu, natto, tempeh, tamari, shoyu, soya yoghurt (from soya)

* sourdough bread (from wheat or rye).

Overall, giving your child a plant-based diet high in fruits and vegetables, which are naturally high in fibre, is much more likely to encourage healthy bacteria. On the other hand, a high meat diet, which, apart from being the primary source of gastrointestinal infections, is more likely to introduce toxic breakdown products as well as slowing down gastrointestinal transit time.

A daily supplement of probiotics

Another way to ensure a good balance of healthy bacteria is to give your child a supplement of probiotics. These supplements are made by culturing bacteria then freeze-drying them into a powder or capsule or in a drink. They are quite delicate organisms so the supplements are best kept in the fridge. When they are swallowed and come into contact with moisture, they come back to life.

Generally, you need to give your child the equivalent of half a billion of each strain of bacteria, which is probably one-quarter or half a teaspoon, but check the dose suggested by the manufacturer (see

Resources for details). For babies and young children, a powder form is best, as this can be mixed with a little expressed breast milk and given from a teaspoon or the end of a dropper, or added to formula in bottle (but add once warmed, as heating will kill the good bacteria).

If you are giving probiotics therapeutically, for example, to reinoculate your child's digestive tract after antibiotics or as part of an anti-infection strategy (for example to get rid of a bout of diarrhoea), your child will need three times the normal amount. These higher levels of probiotics can sometimes result in increased flatulence, at least in the short term. This is not necessarily a bad sign. Sometimes, as less desirable organisms die off, symptoms get worse before they get better.

In summary, to boost your child's immune system:

- **Feed** them antioxidant-rich foods such as sweet potatoes, carrots, kiwi fruits, green leafy vegetables, avocados, fish and broccoli.

- **Give** extra vitamin C when required – the recommended daily dose up to six times a day.

- **Limit** mucus-making foods such as meat, dairy and eggs when your child is congested, and restrict all sugar when they need to fend off any infection.

- **Incorporate** regular exercise into their daily regime.

- **To** boost levels of healthy gut bacteria, feed them a more plant-based diet and include in the diet fermented foods such as yoghurt, cottage cheese, miso, shoyu, sauerkraut and sourdough bread.

- **Give** them a probiotic supplement as a powder or drink if they are unwell or are taking a course of antibiotics, or to treat diarrhoea.

❧

CHAPTER TWENTY-SEVEN

Healthy Food Your Child Will Love

ONCE YOUR CHILD is a year old, there's no reason why they can't eat the same food as the rest of the family. Although there are bound to be dishes they will enjoy more than others, these can easily be incorporated into family mealtimes. And, as they grow older, you can get them involved with food preparation so they can appreciate the satisfaction of a supper that does not come breaded and out of a box in the freezer. You can also appeal to a child's love of colour by actively encouraging them to eat their reds, yellows and oranges as well as their greens. Here are some meal suggestions to provide food for thought.

Breakfast ideas

Mixed wholegrain porridge

Instead of serving up sugar-filled cereals or tasteless instant oat cereals lacking in nutrients, buy wholegrain flakes, such as millet, brown rice, quinoa, oats, barley, buckwheat and/or rye from your local healthfood shop and combine. Make into porridge with water or milk (goat, soya, nut or oat) and stir in chopped-up fruit, such as plums, apricots or bananas and a tablespoon of freshly ground seeds (flax, sunflower, sesame and pumpkin). The fruit gives the porridge a natural sweetness and seeds give a long-lasting energy boost.

Herby corn bread

175g yellow cornmeal
150g live yoghurt
1 egg, beaten
2 tbsp olive oil
1 tsp mixed dried herbs
1½ tsp bicarbonate of soda
½ tsp salt

Preheat the oven to 200°C/390°F/gas 6. Mix the cornmeal, bicarbonate of soda, herbs and salt. Mix the egg with the yoghurt and oil, and pour over the mixture, combining well. Bake in a loaf tin or muffin tray (makes 6) for 15–20 minutes, until golden and firm.

Serve with grilled mushrooms and tomatoes and poached or scrambled egg.

Fruit smoothies

Purée fruit and mixed seeds with live yoghurt for a delicious breakfast in a glass. Serve as a soup with sesame snap 'croutons' (available from most food shops) if you want to serve a healthy drink in the guise of a pudding.

Simple meals

Really easy risotto

Stir fish, chopped hard-boiled egg or meat, with plenty of vegetables into cooked brown rice. You can make a very easy kedgeree this way (using hard-boiled egg, haddock with peas and chopped tomatoes), or try prawns and spring onion.

Alternate rice with a variety of wholegrains such as millet, hulled barley (a better energy source than the more common, polished pearl variety), quinoa or couscous (Belazu make an excellent barley one, if your child is wheat intolerant – available from good supermarkets, delis and healthfood stores).

A rice cooker, particularly one with a steamer tray above, makes this into a one-pot wonder, as you can cook large quantities of rice and simply add your fish and vegetables in the last few minutes to cook or warm through, retaining all the nutrients.

Omelettes

Omelettes make brilliant store cupboard standbys as you can simply add chopped meat, tinned fish or tomatoes and any leftovers. Use free-range eggs (in the UK, Columbus eggs are from chickens fed on flaxseeds and so are incredibly rich in Omega 3 fats). Serve with vegetables or a salad.

Fish cakes

Mix flaked fish (cod, fresh tuna or organic salmon, for example) with mashed sweet potatoes, swede, butternut squash or carrot, instead of or in addition to the usual potato, with added onion. Serve with a sauce of parsley and lemon juice stirred into yoghurt.

Homemade 'nuggets'

White meat or fish fillets or sticks of firm tofu dipped in beaten egg and coated with couscous or breadcrumbs make a good alternative to commercial brands. Bake or grill until crisp and golden. Cut into goujons to make nuggets, for more 'McMeal' appeal. You can even make convincing fish fingers in this way by adding a teaspoon of turmeric to the crumbs, to achieve the lurid orange of the shop-bought variety.

Easy tomato sauce

Add a crushed clove of garlic, a small, finely chopped onion, a handful of cherry tomatoes and a couple of chopped sundried tomatoes to a pan, and lightly sauté in a dribble of olive oil. Add half a can of chopped tomatoes, simmer for 30 minutes and season to taste. This sauce can be easily adapted if you want to add different ingredients such as black olives, roasted peppers and red onion, or basil and pine nuts. It can be stirred into pasta, used as a base in soups and casseroles or served alongside meat, fish, tofu or roasted vegetables.

Easy snacks

Crudités

Chop a variety of raw vegetables – carrots, celery, red and yellow peppers, raw mushrooms, for example – into bite-sized sticks and serve with dips.

- Hummus (easy to make with chickpeas, but also with flageolet or butter beans and red lentils)

- Guacamole

- Tofu blended with a few dollops of tomato salsa

- Pumpkin seed butter (this gruesome-looking green goo tastes delicious and is higher in healthier fats than peanut butter. Available in some healthfood stores or from Higher Nature – see Resources)

- Fish pâté (blend canned fish with silken tofu or cream cheese and lemon juice)

Homemade crisps and chips

Cut pitta bread or corn or flour tortillas into triangles or strips, spray with olive oil, sprinkle with sesame seeds and bake at 230°C/450°F/gas 8 for 4–5 minutes until crisp and golden, to make a healthier alternative to crisps. Roasted potato or sweet potato wedges sprinkled with sesame seeds are delicious snacks served with a dipping sauce.

Stuffed tomatoes and peppers

Cut the tops off raw vegetables or roast peppers at 190°C/375°F/gas 5 for 15 minutes or until soft, remove insides and stuff with:

- hard-boiled egg with mayonnaise

- cottage cheese or mashed tofu

- couscous with baby corn and red pepper

- ratatouille

- mixed pulse salad

- tuna and sweetcorn

- rice salad

- prawn and avocado.

Raw vegetable and pasta or lentil soup

Put any finely chopped vegetables (except root vegetables) in a food processor with a little water and blend well. Add a can of chopped tomatoes or passata and season to taste. Heat gently before serving, with a handful of (precooked) wholemeal pasta or lentils thrown in for a more filling meal. By not cooking the vegetables you preserve more vitamins and enzymes.

Sweet treats

Baked apple slices

Heat sliced apples in a pan over a gentle heat with 1 dessertspoon of butter and 1 dessertspoon of lemon juice, until the fruit is soft and golden. Add sultanas if liked, and sprinkle cinnamon and ginger over the top. Serve on its own or with a drizzle of honey and yoghurt.

Fruit fondue

Dip dried and fresh fruit into fruit yoghurt, stewed fruit compote or lemon curd.

Berry and banana ice lollies

Makes 12 × 50ml lollies
2 ripe bananas
310ml (11fl oz) natural cow/goat/sheep/soya yoghurt
75g (3oz) berries (such as blueberries, blackberries or raspberries)

Blitz the peeled bananas in a blender. Add the fruit and yoghurt and whiz for a minute until the mixture is smooth and the colour even. (Mash the fruits with a fork if you do not have a blender.) Pour the mixture into lolly moulds and drop a stick in each one (or put into a large container to make a frozen yoghurt pudding). Freeze for 1 hour.

Baked apple meringues

Parbake cooking apples with mincemeat spooned in the middle, then top with meringue (whip egg whites with as little caster sugar as possible, until thick and shiny) and flaked almonds. Bake until golden.

Raspberry mousse

Beat 2 egg whites until stiff, then fold into 575ml/1 pint of live raspberry yoghurt. Chill until the mixture has set slightly and serve within an hour of making, with fresh raspberries.

Fruit gums

Instead of fruit pastilles, use a circular cutter to make sweetie shapes out of dried fruit such as apricots, mango pieces or prunes.

Chocolate crispies

Follow a standard crispy recipe, but replace half the quantity of rice crispies with oats, and stir mixed seeds and dried fruit into the mixture. Sweeten with brown rice syrup and use good-quality dark chocolate.

Banana and mixed seed flapjacks

Add a mashed banana to a classic flapjack mixture, sweeten with honey or molasses and sprinkle in some mixed seeds. The texture is much more moist than the traditional version and the consistency more like that of a cake.

References

⁓

Part One

1. C. J. Chuong and E. B. Dawson, 'Zinc and copper levels in premenstrual syndrome', *Fertility and Sterility*, vol. 62 (1994), pp. 313–21

2. R. Bayer, 'Treatment of infertility with vitamin E', *International Journal of Infertility*, vol. 5 (1960), pp. 430–4

3. R. Hakim et al., 'Alcohol and caffeine consumption and decreased fertility', *Fertility and Sterility*, vol. 70, no. 4 (1988), pp. 632–7

4. T. Jensen et al., 'Does moderate alcohol consumption affect fertility? Follow-up study among couples planning first pregnancy', *British Medical Journal*, vol. 317 (1998), pp. 505–10

5. A. Wilcox et al., 'Caffeinated beverages and decreased fertility', *Lancet*, vol. 2 (1988), pp. 1453–5

6. N. Holmberg, *Acta Obstetricia & Gynecologica, Scandinavica*, vol. 50 (1971), pp. 241–6

7. D. Hamilton-Fairley et al., 'Association of moderate obesity with a poor pregnancy outcome in women with polycystic ovary syndrome treated with low dose gonadotrophin', *British Journal of Obstetric Gynaecology*, vol. 99 (1992), pp. 128–31

8. G. Loverro, 'The plasma homocysteine levels are increased in polycystic ovary syndrome', *Gynecology & Obstetrics Investigation*, vol. 53 (2002), pp. 157–62

9. B. V. Sastry and V. E. Janson, 'Depression of human sperm motility by inhibition of enzymatic methylation', *Biochemical Pharmacology*, vol. 32 (1983), pp. 1423–32

10. 'Mom's urinary tract infections increases risk of retardation', *Journal of Family Practice*, vol. 50 (2001), pp. 433–7

11. J. Nevis, unpublished paper (1993), details available from Foresight

12. UK Office for National Statistics. See www.statistics.gov.uk

13. N. Tromans, E. Natamba, J. Jefferies & P. Norman, 'Have national trends in fertility between 1986 and 2006 occurred evenly across England and Wales?', Office of National Statistics, *Population Trends*, vol. 133 (2008), pp. 7–19

14. C. P. West, 'Age and infertility', *British Medical Journal*, vol. 294 (1987), p. 853

15. E. C. Martin, 'Birth intervals and development of nine year olds in Singapore', *IPPF Medical Bulletin* (1978)

16. G. Chamberlain et al., British Birth Surveys 1970: volume one, *The first week of life*, London: Heinemann (1978)

17. 'Average IVF success rates for women aged 40 and under', *Fertility Problems and Treatment – Facts & Figures*, Human Fertilisation & Embryology Authority, published in conjunction with 2006–2007 HFEA *Guide to Infertility*

18. M. Fox, 'Oestrogen mimics,' *Green Network News* (March 1994), pp. 14–15

19. E. Carlsen et al., 'Evidence for decreasing quality of semen during past 50 years', *British Medical Journal*, vol. 305 (1992), pp. 609–12

20. S. Irvine et al., *British Medical Journal*, vol. 312 (1996), pp. 467–71

21. R. M. L. Winston, *Infertility, A Sympathetic Approach*, London: Martin Dunitz Ltd (1986)

22. P. K. Working, 'Male reproductive toxicology: comparison of the human to animal models', *Environmental Health Perspectives*, vol. 77 (1988), pp. 37–44

23. D. M. de Kretser, 'Declining sperm counts', *British Medical Journal*, vol. 312 (1996), pp. 457–8

24. K. Kucheria, R. Saxena & D. Mohan, 'Semen analysis in alcohol dependence syndrome', *Andrologia*, vol. 17 (1985), pp. 558–63 and A. Brzek, 'Alcohol and male fertility' (Preliminary report), *Andrologia*, vol. 19 (1987), pp. 32–6

25. S. Davis & A. Stewart, *Nutritional Medicine*, London: Pan Books (1987), pp. 138–42

26. R. Balarajan & M. McDowall, 'Congenital malformations and agricultural workers', *Lancet* (1983), i: 1112–3

27. ABPI Data Sheet Compendium, 1991–2, compiled by G. Walker, Published by Datapharm Publications, p. 690

28. C. G. Fraga et al., 'Ascorbic acid protects against endogenous oxidative DNA damage in human sperm', *Proceedings of the National Academy of Science*, vol. 88 (1996), pp. 11003–6

29. E. R. Gonzales, 'Sperm swim singly after vitamin C therapy', *Journal of the American Medical Association*, vol. 249 (1983), p. 2747

30. K. C. Srivastava et al., 'Prostaglandin E and 19-hydroxy-prostaglandin E content in the semen of men with normal sperm characteristics, men with abnormal sperm characteristics, vasectomised men and polyzoospermic men', *Danish Medical Bulletin*, vol. 28 (1981)

31. R. Bayer, 'Treatment of infertility with vitamin E', *International Journal of Infertility*, vol. 5 (1960), pp. 430–4

32. R. A. Anderson & M. M. Polansky, 'Dietary chromium deficiency: effect on sperm count and fertility in rats', *Biological Trace Element Research*, vol. 3 (1981), pp. 1–5

33. P. Chanmugam, *Journal of Nutrition*, vol. 114 (1984), p. 2073

34. W. Doyle et al., 'Maternal nutrient intake and birth weight,' *Journal of Human Nutrition and Dietetics*, vol. 2 (1989), pp. 415–22

35. N. I. Ward & D. Bryce-Smith, 'Lead, cadmium and zinc levels in relation to fetal development and abnormalities', (Stillbirths, Spina Bifida and Hydrocephalus), *Heavy Metals in the Environment*, vol. 2 (1993), pp. 280–4

36. L. H. Smith, MD, with J. G. Hattersley, MA, *The Infant Survival Guide: Protecting Your Baby from the Dangers of Crib Death, Vaccines and Other Environmental Hazards*, Petaluma, CA: Smart Publications (2002)

37. H. L. Needleman, 'Lead and neuro psychological deficit', *Low Level Lead Exposure: the clinical implications and current research*, New York: Raven Press (1980), pp. 43–51

38. B. Barnes & S. G. Bradley, *Planning for a Healthy Baby*, London: Vermilion (1994), p. 91

39. Dr J. Mercola, 'What you must know before eating fish', www.mercola.com (2002)

40. S. E. Schober et al., 'Mercury blood levels in U.S. children and women of child-bearing age, 1999-2000', *Journal of the American Medical Association*, vol. 289 (2003), pp. 1667–74

41. Cowdry et al., 'Aluminium in the water causes senile dementia', *Daily Telegraph*, 13 January 1989

42. E. Lodge Rees, 'Aluminium toxicity as indicted by hair analysis', *Journal of Orthomolecular Psychiatry*, vol. 8, no. 1 (1979), pp. 37–43

43. S. Heaton, *Organic Farming, Food Quality and Human Health: A Review of the Evidence*, Bristol: Soil Association (2001)

44. M. Holland, *International Journal of Environmental Studies*, vol. 17 (1981), pp. 67–71

45. P. Lemoine et al., 'Les enfants de parents alcoholiques: anomalies observees a propos de 127 Cas', *Quest Medical*, vol. 25 (1968), pp. 476 –82

46. M. Holland, *International Journal of Environmental Studies*, vol. 17 (1981), pp. 67–71

47. *New Scientist* (August 1985)

48. S. Pieroq et al., 'Withdrawal symptoms in infants with fetal alcohol syndrome', *Journal of Pediatrics*, vol. 90, no. 4 (1977), p. 630

49. D. D. Lewis, 'Alcohol and pregnancy outcome', *Midwives Chronicle & Nursing Notes* (December 1983), pp. 420–3 and E. L. Abel & R. J. Sokol, 'Incidence of fetal alcohol syndrome and economic impact of FAS-related abnormalities', *Drug Alcohol Dependence*, vol. 19 (1987), pp. 51–70

50. A. P. Streissguth, 'Prenatal alcohol-induced brain damage and long-term post natal consequences', *Alcoholism: Clinical & Experimental Research*, vol. 14, no. 5 (1990), pp. 648–9

51. T. Tuornamm, 'The adverse effects of alcohol on reproduction', *Journal of Nutritional and Environmental Medicine*, vol. 6 (1996), pp. 379–91

52. L. Yeh, *Journal of Nutrition*, vol. 114 (1984), p. 2027

53. M. A. Stenchever et al., 'Chromosome breakages in users of marijuana', *American Journal of Obstetrics & Gynecology*, vol. 118 (1974), pp. 106–13

54. M. Brett, 'Cannabis and its effects', talk given at Foresight lecture, Godalming, England, 20 June 2003

55. C. Leuchtenberger et al., 'Effects of marihuana and tobacco smoke on DNA and chromosomal complement in human lung explants', *Nature*, vol. 242 (1973), pp. 403–4 and H. Yager, 'Alveolar cells: depressant effect of cigarette smoke on protein synthesis', *Proc Soc Exp Bio Med*, issue 131, (1969), pp. 147–50

56. L. M. Hellman et al., 'Some factors affecting fetal heart rate', *American Journal of Obstetrics & Gynecology*, vol. 82 (1969), pp. 1055–63

57. M. & A. Wynn, *The Prevention of Handicap of Early Pregnancy Origin*, published by The Foundation for Education and Research in Childbearing, London (1981), pp. 28–33

58. M. Belsey, 'The World Health evidence: the mother is the key to the next generation', *Nutrition and Health*, vol. 9 (1993), pp. 75–80

59. M. & A. Wynn, *The Prevention of Handicap of Early Pregnancy Origin*, published by The Foundation for Education and Research in Childbearing, London (1981), pp. 28–33

60. T. M. Frazier et al., 'Cigarette smoking and prematurity: A predictive study', *American Journal of Obstetrics & Gynecology*, vol. 81 (1961), pp. 988–96

61. J. Golding, 'The consequences of smoking in pregnancy', lecture given to Smoking in Pregnancy conference, organised by the Health Education Authority (February 1994)

62. J. Mercoff et al., 'Effect of food supplementation (WIC) during pregnancy on birthweight', *American Journal of Clinical Nutrition*, vol. 42 (1985), pp. 933–47

63. R. L. Naeye & E. C. Peters, 'Mental development of children whose mothers smoked during pregnancy', *Obstetrics & Gynecology*, vol. 64, no. 4 (1984), pp. 601–7

64. P. Rantakallio et al., 'Maternal smoking during pregnancy and delinquency of the offspring: an association without causation?', *International Journal of Epidemiology*, vol. 21 (1992), pp. 1106–13

65. P. Rantakallio, 'Relationship of maternal smoking to morbidity and mortality of the child up to the age of five', *Acta Paediatrica, Scandinavia*, vol. 67 (1978), pp. 621–31

66. W. Doyle, M. A. Crawford, A. Wynn & S. Wynn, 'The association between maternal diet and birth and birth dimensions', *Journal of Nutritional Medicine*, vol. 1 (1990), pp. 9–17

67. K. R. Niswander & M. Gordon, 'The women and their pregnancies', Washington: US Department of Health, Education and Welfare (1972)

68. A. E. Czeizal, 'Prevention of congenital abnormalities by periconceptual multivitamin supplementation', *British Medical Journal*, vol. 306 (1993), pp. 1645–8

69. W. L. Nelen et al., 'Homocysteine and folate levels as risk factors for recurrent early pregnancy loss', *Obstet Gynecol*, vol. 95, no. 4 (2000), pp. 519–24.

70. T. O. Scholla & W. G. Johnson, 'Folic acid: influence on the outcome of pregnancy', *American Journal of Clinical Nutrition*, vol. 71 (2000), pp. 129–303

71. P. Sanderson, 'Folate bioavailability: Food Standards Agency workshop report', *British Journal of Nutrition*, vol. 90 (2003), pp. 473–9

72. G. Saner, *American Journal of Clinical Nutrition*, vol. 41, no. 5 (1985), pp. 1042

73. R. F. Harrell et al., 'Can nutritional supplements help mentally retarded children? An exploratory study', *Proceedings of the National Academy of Sciences of the United States of America*, vol. 78, no. 1 (1981), pp. 574–8

74. J. Dobbing, *Early Human Development*, vol. 12 (1985), pp. 1–8

75. J. Meyer & Z. F. Kinderheilk, reviewed in *The Prevention of Handicap of Early Pregnancy Origin* by A. & M. Wynn, London: Foundation for Educational Research in Childbearing (1983)

76. 'Painkillers "may boost miscarriage risk"', BBC News, www.bbc.co.uk, 15 August 2003

77. A. Streissguth, 'Aspirin and acetaminophen use by pregnant women and subsequent child IQ and attention decrements', *Teratology*, vol. 35 (1987), pp. 211–19

78. J. Kocisova et al., 'Mutagenicity studies on paracetamol in human volunteers', *Mutation Research*, vol. 209 (1988), pp. 161–5

79. J. E. Zellars & R. F. Gautieri, 'Evaluation of peratogenic potential of codeine sulphate in CF-mice', *Journal of Pharmacology Science*, vol. 66 (1977), pp. 1727–31

80. L. W. D. Weber, 'Benzodiazepines in pregnancy – academical debate or teratogenic risk?', *Biological Research in Pregnancy*, vol. 64 (1985), pp. 151–67

81. C. D. Chambers et al., 'Birth outcomes in pregnant women taking Fluoxetine', *New England Journal of Medicine*, vol. 225 (1996), pp. 1010–15

82. C. G. Smith, 'Reproductive toxicity; hypothalamic-pituitary mechanisms', *American Journal of Industrial Medicine*, vol. 4 (1983), pp. 107–12

83. D. J. P. Barker, 'The fetal and infant origins of adult disease', *British Medical Journal,* vol. 301 (1990), pp. 1111

84. S. E. Vollset et al., 'Plasma total homocysteine, pregnancy complications, and adverse pregnancy outcomes: the Hordaland Homocysteine study', *American Journal of Clinical Nutrition*, vol. 71, no. 4 (2000), pp. 962–8

85. P. de Marco, 'Polymorphisms in genes involved in folate metabolism as risk factors for NTDs', *European Journal of Paediatric Surgery*, supp. 1 (2001), pp. S14–17

86. W. L. Nelen et el., 'Homocysteine and folate levels as risk factors for recurrent early pregnancy loss', *Obstetrics & Gynecology*, vol. 95, no. 4 (2000), pp. 519–24

87. R. Carmi et al., 'Spontaneous abortion – high risk factor for neural tube defects in subsequent pregnancy', *American Journal of Medical Genetics*, vol. 13, no. 55 (1995), p. 512

88. H. Böhles et al., 'Maternal plasma homocysteine, placenta status and docosahexaenoic acid concentration in erythrocyte phospholipids of the newborn', *European Journal of Pediatrics*, vol. 158 (1999), pp. 243–6

89. *US News and World Report*, vol. 106, no. 7 (1989), p. 77

90. J. Braly & R. Hoggan, *Dangerous Grains*, New York: Avery (2002), pp. 28–9

91. U. Erasmus, *Fats That Heal, Fats That Kill*, Burnaby, BC: Alive Books (1993), p. 380

92. Pediatrics Online, vol. 111 (2003), e. 39–44

93. S. F. Olsen & N. J. Secher, 'Low consumption of seafood in early pregnancy as a risk factor for preterm delivery: prospective cohort study', *British Medical Journal*, vol. 324 (2002), pp. 447–50

94. Annual Meeting of the American Psychiatric Association; San Francisco, CA (20 May 2003)

95. F. Safford, Florida International University

96. X. Willet, Harvard (1994)

97. U. Erasmus, *Fats That Heal, Fats That Kill*, Burnaby, BC: Alive Books (1993), p. 112

Part Two

1. D. J. P. Barker, *Mothers, Babies and Diseases in Later Life*, London: BMJ Publishing Group (1994)

2. UK Dietary Reference Values in Pregnancy (Department of Health), *BioMed Newsletter*, no. 18 (1999)

3. R. Cumming et al., 'Calcium intake and fracture risk: results from the study of osteoporotic fractures', *American Journal of Epidemiology*, vol. 145 (1997), pp. 926–34

4. N. Freinkel, 'The honeybee syndrome – implications of the teratogenicity of mannose in rat-embryo culture', *New England Journal of Medicine*, vol. 310, no. 4 (1984), p. 223

5. C. Fisher, 'Nutrition and pregnancy', *BioMed Newsletter*, no. 18 (1999)

6. Ibid.

7. G. Goldenberg, 'The effect of zinc supplementation on pregnancy outcome', *Journal of the American Medical Association*, vol. 274, no. 6 (1995), pp. 4635; M. Richards et al., 'Birth weight and cognitive function in the British 1946 birth cohort: longitudinal population based study', *British Medical Journal*, vol. 7280, no. 322 (2001), pp. 199–203

8. P. Cook, 'March chicken survey', Microbiological Safety Division, Food Standards Agency (1996)

9. M. Klebanoff et al., 'Maternal serum paraxanthine, a caffeine metabolite, and the risk of spontaneous abortion', *New England Journal of Medicine*, no. 341 (1999), pp. 1639–44, 1688–9

10. G. M. Shaw et al., 'Maternal periconceptional use of multivitamins and reduced risk for conotruncal heart defects and limb deficiencies among offspring', *American Journal of Medical Genetics*, vol. 59, no. 4 (1995), pp. 536–45

11. Ibid., *American Journal of Epidemiology*, no. 146 (1997), pp. 134–41

12. S. Rautava et al., 'Probiotics during pregnancy and breast-feeding might confer immunomodulatory protection against atopic disease in the infant', *Journal of Allergy & Clinical Immunology*, vol. 109 (2002), pp. 119–21

13. Annual Meeting of the American Psychiatric Association; San Francisco, USA (20 May 2003)

14. B. Pickard, *Nausea and Vomiting in Pregnancy* booklet
15. C. Zhang et al., 'Vitamin C and the risk of pre-eclampsia – results from dietary questionnaire and plasma assay', *Epidemiology*, no. 13 (2002), pp. 409–16; L. C. Chappell et al., 'Effect of antioxidants on the occurrence of pre-eclampsia in women at increased risk: a randomised trial', *Lancet*, vol. 354, no. 9181 (1999), pp. 810–16; M. Wachstein & L. Graffeo, 'Influence of vitamin B6 on the incidence of pre-eclampsia', *Obstetrics & Gynaecology*, no. 8 (1956), p. 177; F. B. Pipkin, 'Risk factors for pre-eclampsia', *New England Journal of Medicine*, vol. 344, no. 12 (2001), editorial; *Obstetrics & Gynaecology*, no. 96 (2000), pp. 38–44
16. M. Richards et al., 'Birth weight and cognitive function in the British 1946 birth cohort: longitudinal population based study', *British Medical Journal*, vol. 7280, no. 322 (2001), pp. 199–203
17. Conference Review, *Nutrition and Health*, vol. 8 (1992), pp. 45–55
18. J. F. Clapp et al., 'Beginning regular exercise in early pregnancy: effect on feto-placental growth', *American Journal of Obstetrics & Gynecology*, no. 183 (2000), pp. 1484–8
19. APA Monitor, vol. 30, no. 9 (1999)
20. M. R. Sable & D. S. Wilkinson, 'Impact of perceived stress, major life events and pregnancy attitudes on low birth weight', *Family Planning Perspectives*, vol. 32, no. 6 (2000), pp. 288–94
21. J. F. Clapp et al., 'Beginning regular exercise in early pregnancy: effect on feto-placental growth', *American Journal of Obstetrics & Gynecology*, no. 183 (2000), pp. 1484–8

Part Three

1. G. Golding et al., 'Childhood cancer, intramuscular vitamin K and pethidine given during labour', *British Medical Journal*, vol. 305 (1992), pp. 241–346
2. American Dietetic Association, 'Promotion of breastfeeding', *Journal of American Dietetic Association*, vol. 97 (1997), pp. 662–6
3. M. Martin, 'Is DHA the secret of breast milk's success?' *WorldNetDaily.com* (2002)
4. F. Martinez, *American Journal of Clinical Nutrition*, vol. 41, no. 3 (1985), p. 969
5. C. Kunz, *International Journal for Vitamin & Nutrient Research*, vol. 54, no. 141 (1984)
6. W. Craig, *Nutrition Reports International*, vol. 30, no. 4 (1984), p. 1003
7. J. Armstrong et al., 'Breastfeeding and lowering the risk of childhood obesity', *Lancet*, vol. 359, no. 9322 (2002), pp. 2003–4
8. 'Breastfeeding step by step', The National Childbirth Trust information sheet
9. Collaborative Group on Hormonal Factors in Breast Cancer, 'Breast cancer and breastfeeding: collaborative reanalysis of individual data from 47 epidemiological studies in 30 countries, including 50,302 women with breast cancer and 96,973 women without the disease', *Lancet*, vol. 360 (2002), pp. 187–96
10. S. Roberts, *British Journal of Nutrition*, vol. 53, no. 1 (1985)

11. L. Styslinger, *American Journal of Clinical Nutrition*, vol. 41, no. 1 (1985), p. 21

12. L. Byerley, *American Journal of Clinical Nutrition*, vol. 41, no. 3 (1985), p. 666

13. Annual Meeting of the American Psychiatric Association; San Francisco, USA (20 May 2003)

14. Z. Weizman et al., 'Efficacy of herbal tea preparation in infantile colic', *Journal of Pediatrics*, vol. 122, no. 4 (1993), pp. 650–2

15. M. Kailliomäki et al., 'Probiotics in primary prevention of atopic disease: a randomised placebo-controlled trial', *Lancet*, vol. 357 (2001), pp. 1076–9

16. Feature quoting statistics from the London Bills of Mortality 1760–1834 and Reports of the Registrar General 1836–96, as compiled by Alfred Wallace, *The Wonderful Century* (1898); *Campaign against Fraudulent Medical Research Newsletter*, vol. 2, no. 3 (1995), pp. 5–13

17. P. A. Patriarca, 'Polio outbreaks: a tale of torment', *Lancet*, vol. 344 (1994), pp. 630–1

18. J. Walene, *Immunization: The Reality Behind the Myth*, Massachusetts: Bergen & Garvey (1988)

19. *Clinical Infectious Diseases*, Centers for Disease Control and Prevention (CDC) (February 1992), pp. 568–79

20. M. Gaier & D. Gaier, 'Thimerosal in childhood vaccines, neurodevelopment disorders and heart disease in the United States', *Journal of American Physicians and Surgeons* (2003)

Part Four

1. L. H. Smith & J. G. Hattersley, 'Victory over crib death', *Townsend Letter for Doctors and Patients* (Aug/Sept 2000 issue)

2. J. Braly & R. Hoggan, *Dangerous Grains*, New York: Avery (2002), p. 24

3. The Vegetarian Society of the United Kingdom, website, September 2003

4. Gallup: The Realeat Survey 1997, 'Changing attitudes to meat consumption', Haldane Foods (1997)

5. P. Sanderson et al., 'Folate bioavailability: UK Food Standards Agency workshop report', *British Journal of Nutrition*, vol. 90 (2003), pp. 473–9

6. A. Hoffer, 'Vitamin B3 dependent child', *Schizophrenia*, vol. 3 (1971), pp. 107–13

7. I. Colquhon & S. Bunday, 'A lack of essential fatty acids as a possible cause of hyperactivity in children', *Medical Hypotheses*, vol. 7 (1981), pp. 673–9

8. B. O'Reilly, Hyperactive Children's Support Group Conference (June 2001), UK

9. M. D. Boris & F. S. Mandel, *Annals of Allergy*, vol. 72 (1994), pp. 462–8

10. R. J. Theil, 'Nutrition based interventions for ADD and ADHD', *Townsend Letter for Doctors and Patients* (April 2000), pp. 93–5

11. A. R. Swain et al., 'Salicylates, oligoantigenic diet and behaviour', *Lancet*, vol. 2, no. 8445 (1985), pp. 41–2

12. R. J. Prinz et al. 'Dietary correlates of hyperactive behaviour in children', *Journal of Consulting Clinical Psychology*, vol. 48 (1980), pp. 760–9

13. L. Langseth & J. Dowd, 'Glucose tolerance and hyperkinesis', *Food & Cosmetic Toxicology*, vol. 16 (1978), p. 129

14. N. I. Ward et al., 'The influence of the chemical additive Tartrazine on the zinc status of hyperactive children – a double-blind placebo controlled study', *Journal of Nutritional Medicine*, vol. 1 (1990), pp. 51–7

15. J. R. Ringsdorf et al., 'Sucrose, neutrophilic phagocytosis and resistance to disease', *Dental Survey* (December 1976), pp. 46–8

16. N. I. Ward, 'Assessment of clinical factors in relation to child hyperactivity', *Journal of Nutritional and Environmental Medicine*, vol. 7 (1997), pp. 333–42

17. N. I. Ward, 'Hyperactivity and a previous history of antibiotic usage', *Nutrition Practitioner*, vol. 3, no. 3 (2001), p. 12

18. M. F. Bernet et al., 'Lactobacillus acidophilus LA1 binds to cultured human intestinal cell lines and inhibits cell attachment and cell invasion by enterovirulent bacteria', *Gut*, vol. 35 (1994), pp. 483–9

19. H. Majamaa & E. Isolaui, 'Probiotics: a novel approach in the management of food allergy', *Journal of Allergy & Clinical Immunology*, vol. 99 (1997), pp. 179–85

Resources

∾

Useful contacts

Baby mattress covers – Babesafe produces slip-on covers for babies' mattresses to protect against any harmful fumes or elements being released from the synthetic ingredients in the mattress that may contribute to cot death. In the UK, these mattresses are sold by many online retail outlets including Patient UK (see www.patient.co.uk). Outside the UK, visit www.babesafe.com for stockists.

Cranial osteopathy – the Sutherland Society can put you in touch with a practitioner in your area who can, via gentle manipulation, help to realign subtle imbalances in both babies and adults. Website: www.cranial.org.uk

Foresight, the pre-conceptual care charity, can provide help and support and refer you to a local practitioner to help you prepare for pregnancy or address any previous reproductive problems. Foresight, 3 Lower Queens Road, Clevedon, North Somerset BS21 6LX. Tel: 01275 878953. Website: www.foresight-preconception.org.uk

Institute for Optimum Nutrition (ION) runs courses including a homestudy course and a three-year Nutritional Therapists Diploma course. It also has a directory of nutritional therapists throughout the UK. ION, Avalon House, 72 Lower Mortlake Road, Richmond TW9 2JY.
Tel: 020 8614 7800. Website: www.ion.ac.uk

La Leche League is a nationwide network that provides mother-to-mother support on breast feeding. PO Box 29, West Bridgford, Nottingham NG2 7NP.
Tel: 0845 120 2918. Website: www.laleche.org.uk

National Childbirth Trust (NCT) has a national network of teachers to provide ante-natal preparation, post-natal support and advice on breast feeding. NCT, Alexandra House, Oldham Terrace, Acton, London W3 6NH.
Tel: 0300 330 0700. Website: www.nct.org.uk

Natural family planning is, as the name suggests, a completely natural method of birth control and pregnancy planning that's 97 per cent reliable. Classes run worldwide. For details see: www.fertilityuk.org

Or read: *A Manual of Natural Family Planning* by A.M. Flynn and M. Brooks, published by Thorsons/HarperCollins, London (1990)

Fertility Awareness and Natural Family Planning by Dr Elizabeth Clubb and Jane Kinght, published by David & Charles, UK (1996).

Vaccinations – BabyJabs is a London-based private clinic offering single-dose vaccinations for babies and children. Tel: 020 7631 0090. Website: www.babyjabs.co.uk

Nutrition consultations

For a personal consultation with Susannah Lawson, call: 07960 020538 or visit www.susannah-lawson.co.uk

Nutrition Consultations

For a personal referral by Patrick Holford to a nutritional therapist in your area, visit www.patrickholford.com and select 'consultations' for an immediate online referral. This service gives details on whom to see in the UK as well as internationally. If there is no one available near by you can always do an online assessment – see below.

Nutrition Assessment Online

You can have your own personal health and nutrition assessment online using my 100% Health Check. This gives you a personalised assessment of your current health, and what you most need to change in order to feel great. Visit www.patrickholford.com and go to 'free on-line assessment.'

Vitamin and mineral supplements

The following companies produce good-quality supplements that we ourselves use in practice.

BioCare produces a wide range of supplements for adults, pregnant women and children, including essential fatty acids (GLA, DHA, EPA), children's probiotics and multivitamins. Tel: 0121 433 3727. Website: www.biocare.co.uk

The Patrick Holford range of supplements – which includes an Optimum Nutrition pack for before, during and after pregnancy, and Chewable Essential Omegas for Children – is available from Holland and Barrett and Totally Nourish. Website: www.totallynourish.com.

Solgar manufactures a wide range of nutritional and herbal supplements including essential fats, children's vitamins and pregnancy formulas. Available in any good healthfood shop. Contact Solgar on 014422 890355 for your nearest supplier.

Food and drink

Babynat organic formula milk for babies.
Website: www.babynat.co.uk

Brita Water Filters make inexpensive jug water filters for reducing toxic metal content in tap water. Tel: 0844 742 4900.
Website: www.brita.net/uk

Columbus are free-range eggs that are rich in essential fats. Stocked by most large supermarkets. Website: www.columbuseggs.co.uk

Fresh Water Filter Company provide main-attached water-filtering units. Tel: 020 8558 7495. Website: www.freshwaterfilter.com

Hipp ready prepared baby foods, available from healthfood shops and major supermarkets. Website: www.hipp.co.uk

Longwood Farm sells organic meat, dairy and other fresh produce by mail order. Tel: 01638 717 120. Website: www.longwoodfarm.co.uk

Organic fruit and vegetable box delivery scheme – contact the Soil Association for details of suppliers operating in your area.
Tel: 0117 314 5000. Website: www.soilassociation.org.uk

Organix ready prepared baby foods. Website: www.organix.com

Nanny Goat baby formula milk, distributed by Vitacare.
Website: www.vitacare.co.uk

The Vegetarian Society provides information and advice to the public. Tel: 0161 925 2000. Website: www.vegsoc.org

Relaxation

T'ai chi – for more information and details of classes in your area, contact: The London School of T'ai Chi Chuan and Traditional Health Resources, LSTCC c/o 30 Arundel Gardens, London W11 2LB. Tel: 020 8566 1677. Website: www.londontaichi.org.uk
or
Taoist T'ai Chi Society of Great Britain. Website: www.taoist.org.uk

Also try your local alternative health centres or healthfood shops for details of local classes and check in the Yellow Pages under sports clubs and associations, complementary therapies or martial arts or visit www.taichiunion.com.

Yoga – for more information and details of a yoga school or teacher in your area, contact:
The British Wheel of Yoga. Tel: 01529 306 851.
Website: www.bwy.org.uk
or
Iyengar Yoga Institute. Tel: 020 7624 3080. Website: www.iyi.org.uk

Psychocalisthenics is an excellent exercise system that takes less than 20 minutes a day, develops strength, suppleness and stamina, and generates vital energy. The best way to learn it is to do Psychocalisthenics Training. For further information, visit www.patrickholford.com. Also available from this website is the book *Master Level Exercise: Psychocalistenics*, and the *Psychocalisthenics* CD and DVD.

Laboratory testing

Homocysteine

Yorktest Laboratories produce a home kit where you can take your own pin-prick blood sample and return it to the lab for analysis. If your homocysteine level is high, full instructions are provided to help you reduce it. At the time of going to press, the test costs £75. Tel: 0800 458 2052. Website: www.yorktest.com

Food or chemical allergy tests

YorkTest sell a home-test kit for food and chemical allergies that requires a pin-prick blood sample. Visit www.yorktest.com for more information and prices.

Genova Diagnostics screen for food and chemical allergies, but require a blood sample to be professionally taken for testing. Call 020 8336 7750 for more information. Website: www.gdx.uk.net

Hair mineral analysis, to determine any presence of toxic metal, can be arranged via a nutritional therapist.

Further reading

Lucy Burney, *Boost Your Child's Immune System*, London: Piatkus 2001.

Dr Adam Carey & Collette Harris, *PCOS: A Women's Guide to Dealing with Polycystic Ovary Syndrome*, London: Thorsons 2000.

Barbara Cousins, *Cooking Without* (wheat and dairy-free recipes), London: HarperCollins 2000.

A. M. Flynn & A. Brooks, *A Manual of Natural Family Planning*, London: Thorsons/HarperCollins 1990.

Patrick Holford & Judy Ridgway, *The Optimum Nutrition Cookbook*, London: Piatkus 1999.

Patrick Holford, *Optimum Nutrition for the Mind* (for more information on nutritional strategies to help ADHD, autism, Down's syndrome and other mental health problems in both adults and children), London: Piatkus 2003.

Patrick Holford & James Braly, *The Homocysteine Solution*, London: Piatkus 2012.

Patrick Holford, *Natural High Chill*, London: Piatkus 2003.

Walene James, *Immunization – Reality Behind the Myth*, Greenwood Press 1995.

Lynne McTaggart, *The Vaccination Bible*, London: HarperCollins 2000.

Neil Z. Miller, *Are Vaccines Safe and Effective?*, New Atlantean Press 2003.

Dian Shepperson Mills & Mike Vernon, *Endometriosis, a Key to Healing Through Nutrition*, London: HarperCollins 2002.

Mark and Angela Stengler, *Your Vital Child* (the ultimate resource for using food, vitamins, herbs and other natural methods to make your children the healthiest they can be), Rodale 2001, available from Amazon.

www.wddty.co.uk – the website for What Doctors Don't Tell You

Index

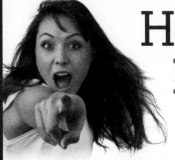

How 100% Healthy are you?

"I thought I was a healthy person. I did the online report. I feel absolutely fantastic. It's changed my life. It's amazing." Karen S

Karen before
36%

Karen after
86%

D	C	B	A
NOT GOOD	AVERAGE	REASONABLY HEALTHY	HEALTHY

YOU CAN wake up full of energy, with a clear mind and balanced mood, never gain weight and stay disease free. Having worked with over 60,000 people We know what changes are going to most rapidly transform how you feel. The **100% Health Programme** is the most comprehensive and genuinely effective way of taking a step towards 100% health.

Your **FREE Health Check** is the first step to receiving your **100% Health Programme** (£24.95), the ultimate on-line personal health profile, that shows you exactly what your perfect diet and daily supplement programme is, and which simple lifestyle changes will make the biggest difference.

You receive:

✔ A full Set of Results on your body systems and processes

✔ In-depth Report on you & your health

✔ Your Perfect Recipes and Menu Plan

✔ Your own Library of Special Reports

✔ Full Lifestyle Analysis inc:
 • Exercise • Stress • Sleep • Pollution

✔ Your Action Plan & Personal Supplement Programme;

✔ PLUS optional weekly support and guidance from Patrick;

✔ Free Reassessment to chart your progress, month by month

✔ Your questions answered by Patrick himself, plus all the benefits of membership

BEGIN YOUR **FREE** HEALTH CHECKUP NOW
Go to **www.patrickholford.com**

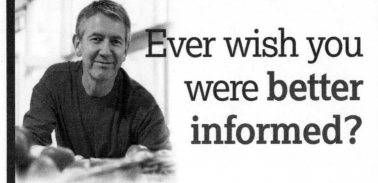